Soulful C

LIVING *alongside* CANCER

CHRISTINE KEEP

Copyright © 2024

All rights reserved. This book or any portion thereof may not be reproduced or used in any manner whatsoever without express written permission of the author except for the use of brief quotations in a book review.

Printed in Australia

First Printing 2024

ISBN: 978-0-6453760-8-1

White Light Publishing

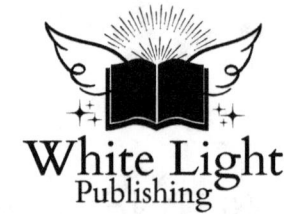

www.whitelightuniversal.com.au

This book is dedicated to:

My beautiful husband, Rod, the hero of this book, whose strength, determination and positive mindset never cease to amaze me;

My daughter, Kate, my heart & soul, always my champion and my voice of reason; and

To all those who have had cancer touch their lives.

TABLE OF CONTENTS

Introduction	1
Part I: Cancer Has Entered Our Lives	3
Chapter One: The Rollercoaster	4
Chapter Two: The Diagnosis	20
Chapter Three: The Treatment Begins	27
Chapter Four: The Holiday Odyssey	37
Chapter Five: The Memories We Made	42
Chapter Six: The Past Twelve Months	51
PART II: My Personal Journey	55
The First Few Days & Weeks	57
Keep Your Chin Up	61
Telling Family and Friends	64
Planning for the Future	67
Our Family Photo Shoot	70
Life On Hold	72
My Darkest Days	75
The Journey	78
My Anger at Rod	80
Support Networks	83
Moving Through Fear	86
Body Changes & Sexual Intimacy	89
Spiritual Beliefs & Complimentary Therapies	93
Our First Holiday	98
Rod's Perspective	101
The Power of Positive Mindset	110
Our Relationship & My Own Self Care	113
In Conclusion: Who Am I Now?	120
Acknowledgments	123
About the Author	124

INTRODUCTION

If you are reading this book, there's a chance that you or someone you know or love, has a cancer diagnosis, and perhaps like we were, you may be wanting to make sense of this new reality and are searching for ways to cope.

If you are at the start of this journey, all I can say is hold on, it can be an overwhelming ride. But through this book, I hope to share with you that it can also be a time of growth and deep reflection; that it is possible to live your life alongside a cancer diagnosis and move through the shock and trauma to a place of acceptance and be able to live completely in the moment. If you are well into this journey, then I hope you find that our experience helps to support and encourage you to navigate your own way through this.

I do talk about my spiritual and holistic beliefs in this book, which if you come from a scientific viewpoint, you may feel these are irrelevant. But through my experience as a counsellor and as someone who has experienced trauma myself, I have learned that having faith and belief in something is paramount to overcoming difficulty and enables us to keep moving forward. I am a big believer in an integrated medical and holistic approach, especially when it comes to a cancer diagnosis. In my perspective, the aim is to create a combination of the right energetic and mindset conditions to support the many medical treatments available to us.

As a deeply spiritual person, I believe in the power of the Universe, signs from spirit and the connection to my own higher self. I love the appearance of rainbows; they are my sign from the Universe that I am going to be okay. No matter what adversity I encounter, the appearance of a rainbow invites an opportunity for spiritual growth and self-reflection. I find them comforting and uplifting, a colorful conduit between this life here on Earth and our link to the Universe. Whenever I see them, I immediately feel calm and supported.

When my husband, Rod, was diagnosed with cancer, my world suddenly felt like it was spinning out of control. I never believed this could happen to us and life as I knew it changed in a moment, leaving me wondering how I would find the strength to get through this. If anyone had told me prior to December 2022 that I would be writing a book about my husband's cancer diagnosis, I would have thought that absurd. But here I am sharing this chapter of our lives with you.

To understand both my and Rod's journey, I have written this memoir in two parts. Through part one I share our experience that brings us to the place where we are today. In part two, I share a reflection of my own journey and spiritual growth, as we continue to navigate our life alongside a rare and aggressive cancer - Cardiac Angiosarcoma.

I write of our personal experiences and how I moved from fear and despair; to acceptance and living completely in the present moment through mindfulness practices, positive mindset and my own spiritual beliefs. As a counsellor, somatic trauma therapist and holistic wellness practitioner my life was filled with supporting others, and I have extensive training in many therapies and was no stranger to self-reflection and working on my own growth - I thought I was in a pretty good place in my life.

All that changed the moment Rod was diagnosed with cancer. I went on a rollercoaster of emotions, and I started to question everything I thought I knew about myself. I had to face the shadow of my soul, my fears, and the parts of myself that I didn't want to share with anyone, let alone with you, the reader of this book. However, I feel it beneficial not only for my own healing but also for you, the reader, to be completely authentic and vulnerable with you.

My hope is that you find some comfort and connection as you read this book, that everything you may be feeling or experiencing is all a part of the grief and trauma process and that you are stronger than you give yourself credit for.

Much love - Christine

Part I

CANCER HAS ENTERED OUR LIVES

We are at the start of a journey, where it leads is unknown, but I have faith that you will always be by my side.

CHAPTER ONE: THE ROLLERCOASTER

"Rod, you have a suspicious mass in your chest. It looks like it's attached to your heart."

These words will be ingrained in my soul forever. I never expected cancer to affect my husband. We've had friends and family die from cancer, but not once did it enter my head that one day this would be Rod. The reason I called this chapter *The Rollercoaster* is because that is exactly what life feels like, all you can do is hold on, scream when you must, and ride it to the end.

But before I start with our journey, I would like to share with you who we are as a couple and what our life was like before this nightmare began.

Rod and I are what we call a "his and hers mixed family." We have both been married before and Rod has two adult children Michael and Melissa. I have an adult daughter, Kate, from my previous marriage. We have grandchildren whom we love dearly. We are what I would consider a standard middle class, working couple. Rod works as a contract manager mainly in the power industry (power stations) for a multinational engineering company and I am a counsellor and holistic therapist in private practice.

We live in a beautiful country town in the southwest of Western Australia called Collie, surrounded by trees and some of the most amazing blue lakes you will ever find. We had worked for many years in various states in Australia, so I was happy when we could finally return home to Western Australia and settle in this beautiful earthy town. We had just sold our other home in Mandurah, Western Australia, deciding that Collie would be the town where we would like to retire to, and like most other couples, we had dreams and hopes for the future, especially for our retirement, which was looming up on us quickly. We are a pretty strong team together; our disagreements are minor, and we don't let our differences of opinions or lifestyles affect how we feel about each other. Rod is passionate about his football which in Australia is called "Aussie Rules," along with fishing and cricket. I love all things spiritual; my crystal and Tibetan sound bowls, my sound healing gong that I affectionately named Lola, my oracle cards, incense and candles and I spend a lot of time in nature, self-reflection and cloud gazing - my favourite - as my way of meditation.

I would describe both of us as hard workers, each passionate about what we do and neither of us are strangers to trauma. Rod lost his mother when he was fifteen, and as the middle of five boys, he and his two older brothers helped their father raise the two younger siblings. We affectionately refer to them as the Keep boys, and like most brothers they used to fight and argue but are fiercely protective of each other should someone else criticize them. Rod's brothers are a huge part of his life and I love how hard they work to stay connected as a family. Losing his mum so young and with so many in the family meant that there wasn't much time to be able to process emotions, and as such Rod is what I would describe as an internaliser, rarely sharing his true feelings, preferring to work things out in his own way the best he can and to just get on with life.

I grew up in what I call a normal household, if you can call any household normal, with my mother, father, sister and brother. We emigrated to Australia in 1972 from the United Kingdom. I was bullied at school and never really felt like I fit in; I had to work hard to be accepted. Having experienced an unhappy and unhealthy marriage in my early twenties, I was passionate about ensuring that my daughter would not grow up in an environment where she felt unsafe, or one filled with conflict. I love horses, but in my early thirties and only six months after recovering from cervical cancer, I had a traumatic riding accident which resulted in a head injury and nearly cost me my life. I had always been a spiritual person, talking to imaginary friends who I thought would go away when I grew up (they never did), but it was the experience of my riding accident that changed the way I view life, death and our connection to the Universe. Spirituality became a bigger part of my life, and I was not afraid to show this side of myself to the world. I would describe myself as an externaliser, preferring to air my thoughts and process them through self-reflection and conversation. So here we have Rod, the internaliser, and me, the externaliser, who are faced with a massive blow and suddenly we must work extremely hard together to navigate this rollercoaster we have now boarded.

July 2022

Our nightmare began when Rod developed pericarditis. We had been away for the weekend at Rod's eldest brother Ken's farm, celebrating his 70th birthday. It was a wonderful weekend that we shared with Rod's brothers, Ken, Gary, and Shane, along with their partners, a couple of relatives and Ken's children. A small affair but one which gave us the opportunity to laugh, reminisce and come together as a family. July is winter in Australia, and it was cold and wet, so we spent most of the weekend inside by the roaring fire or walking through the rain to inspect Ken's dams where the other Keep boys would try to poach the marron that live in there. Marron is a freshwater crustacean and whilst I don't particularly like them, the boys all love them.

Throughout the weekend, I noticed that Rod was very tired, and when we went to bed at night he kept complaining of heartburn. The boys like to have a few drinks when they get together, but I noticed Rod wasn't drinking like he would normally. He struggled to sleep due to the pain in his chest and was uncomfortable the whole weekend. He kept taking heartburn medication, but I wondered whether he was coming down with a cold or flu, especially as he had been out in the rain and cold air a fair bit that weekend. It's always in the back our minds that Rod's mum died of a heart attack at 38 years of age, so I get nervous whenever Rod talks about pain in his chest.

By the time we returned home on the Sunday night, Rod had developed a cough, and I noticed his breathing was heavier than normal. He tried to sleep but the pain kept him awake most of the night, and eventually he propped up the bed so that he could be inclined, which he said made the pain easier. I was uneasy about this and suggested I should take him to the hospital, but he decided he would see how he felt in the morning. Rod's not a person to complain about how he's feeling and finds it difficult to share what is going on with him, so when he said he would be okay, I believed him. Reassured that he would let me know, I managed to get some sleep, unaware just how much pain he was in.

When I woke up in the morning, I could see he was in considerable pain. I wanted to take him straight to the hospital, but he decided he wanted to see his own doctor instead. I remember thinking, *I wonder if it's his heart?*

Rod is a very independent person and not easy to convince when it comes to seeking medical assistance. He drove himself to the doctor while I went to work, but a short time later I got a phone call that the doctor had picked up something on an ECG and he wanted Rod to go straight to the hospital. The doctor wanted to call an ambulance, but Rod told him I was only around the corner and the hospital was less than two minutes away, and I would take him. I went straight to pick him up and took him to our local emergency department. After a few tests, and what seemed to be an agonizing wait, they diagnosed pericarditis (inflammation of the sac around the heart) which meant a hospital stay for a couple of days to get him started on medication and bring his pain under control.

I'm known to be very intuitive, and at the time I was thinking that this was just the start of something bigger and that maybe they were missing something. Rod had worked most of his career in power stations and although he had been extremely careful with safety, there was asbestos in many of the facilities he had worked in. We had lost friends and my father to mesothelioma (an asbestos related cancer), and this has always weighed heavily on my mind whenever Rod developed anything to do with this chest, be that a cough or infection. My fear was that this was the start of mesothelioma. When I mentioned this to the doctors in the hospital, they reassured us that it was pericarditis and that he would start to feel better in a week or so, once the medication kicked in.

I went home that night, upset that my husband was in hospital a street over from our house; I could see the hospital from my lounge window. I couldn't shake the feeling that this was something more, they were missing something, and when one of Rod's colleagues dropped in to see how I was doing, I told him how uneasy I was feeling. I remember standing at the window looking at the hospital with such a sadness hanging over me, picturing my husband in there, in pain, and wondering where this journey would take us.

Rod was released from hospital the next afternoon and he started to improve over the following week. I thought to myself, maybe my fears were unwarranted and that this was something that could be easily treated. I did question how he contracted pericarditis in the first place, but no one could give us those answers.

Everything was starting to settle down, until he stopped taking the medication. Within a week he was back in hospital, this time diagnosed with pneumonia. Again, my soul was feeling very uneasy, and the heaviness was starting to creep back in. Listening to the doctors, they assured us there was nothing to be concerned about on the chest x-ray other than the pneumonia, but they did want him to see a cardiologist to make sure the pericarditis hadn't done any damage to his heart. Once again, he was to stay in hospital, this time for a few days. This felt completely out of the norm for us, Rod doesn't get sick often, so having him in hospital was a shock. After he was released, it took him the better part of a month to recover before he could return to working on site. He had never had that amount of time away from his workplace before, so this was something new for him. He started working from home a little bit more and reduced his hours on site so that he could rest and recover.

August 2022

Rod's appointment with the cardiologist went smoothly. They conducted several tests, along with an external ultrasound. She told us there was no damage to the heart and that everything was okay. Rod still had a nagging cough, which we didn't give much thought to thinking this was just a hangover from the pneumonia, and a follow up was scheduled for the end of October, just to be sure. Life was starting to feel more normal, and I tried to put my fears behind me.

We got on with our lives, excited about the upcoming months. We had lots of plans for the rest of the year, but I noticed Rod was still a little breathless and had this strange cough. I noticed it more when he was on the phone; I could hear him almost suck his breath in as he talked, and I would hear him cough in the bathroom trying to clear his throat. I would mention this to him, but he dismissed it as nothing to worry about. He was also still sleeping slightly inclined in bed, which I found unusual and triggering as my father used to sleep upright to relieve his pain. It brought back all those painful memories of watching him deteriorate. Although Rod was back at work full time, he was coming home very tired and falling asleep on the couch before dinner. This wasn't the Rod I knew, and we put it down to his body taking time to heal - but I still had the niggling feeling that something wasn't quite right.

August - September 2022

We celebrated my 60th birthday with family, and my good friend Vicki flew over from the eastern states for the occasion. Vicki had moved there the previous Christmas and I missed her dearly, so I was excited that she was flying in. We booked an apartment for the three of us on the canals in Mandurah and we had dinner at a restaurant close by with our dearest friends; Kate, her husband Kev; and our granddaughters, Layla and Hannah. Rod, although still tired, was doing okay. We spent a few wonderful days together and my heart was filled with gratitude that I had so many loving people in my life. My fears were starting to ease slightly, and both of us were very much looking forward to the rest of the year. We were starting to put the last few months behind us.

September saw us taking a trip to Exmouth to celebrate our son-in-law, Kev's, 40th birthday. We got to swim with a whale shark on The Ningaloo Reef; a bucket list item for both of us, and the highlight of our year. We spent days at the beach, snorkeling in the pristine waters along that coastline and enjoying our evenings in the caravan park, sharing meals with Kate, Kev and his family. This will be one of the memories I will treasure forever. For years, we had been dreaming of doing just this and finally it had become a reality. I was happy, Rod was happy. After our break, we returned to work and Rod had a busy and hectic few months ahead, so we knew that by Christmas we would be very much looking forward to some more time away.

October 2022

As the month rolled on, we found ourselves back in Northcliffe at Rod's brother Ken's house, to celebrate the wedding of Rod's niece. It was such a beautiful weekend, once again spent with family and friends, although we knew the upcoming appointment with the cardiologist was looming and I could still hear the breathlessness in Rod's voice. He was still sleeping slightly inclined, and I tried not to give that too much thought. I kept reasoning with myself, *it's early days and he has had a lot to cope with health wise these last few months.*

We were in the planning stages of our Christmas trip to South Australia with our friends, Matt and Kay, and their children, Noah and Indi. We were taking our caravans and roof top boats with us. There was much to plan and the closer it got to the final part of the year, the more excited we became.

The October appointment with the cardiologist finally arrived. I thought this was just going to be a routine follow up and I was stunned when Rod mentioned to her about the niggling cough, his breathlessness and a tightness in his chest. He hadn't spoken to me about the tightness in his chest, although his brother, Ken, later told me he had mentioned it to him. I knew he was still a little breathless, but this tightness was something that sideswiped me. She arranged for him to have a CT scan to see what was going on. Unfortunately, this scan couldn't be arranged until the second week of December, some eight weeks later. She didn't seem that concerned as she felt that there was still nothing to worry about. Once again, I tried to push down that dark feeling that something was coming and wasn't going to be good. I often reflect, if they had undertaken a CT scan in July when the pericarditis and pneumonia started instead of just a chest x-ray, would we be where we are today, and I wouldn't be writing this book? But you know what they say about hindsight, so all we could do now was move forward - the past was the past.

November 2022

We were blessed to have a new puppy join our lives, a Cavoodle, who we named Ben. He certainly wasn't on our radar. We had lost one of our dogs, Lucy, a couple of years earlier and even though our big boy dog, Bodhi, was lonely after she died, I didn't feel ready to bring another puppy into our lives just yet. But fate plays a different tune.

Rod had come home one Friday evening and mentioned that there was Bichon Friese crossed with Shit Zhu puppies advertised for sale in the local paper. At first, I said no, I don't want a puppy yet. We had agreed that at the end of next year we would be ready to start looking, but this year was supposed to be about us taking lots of short trips, travelling with our caravan. But curiosity got the better of me and I started searching for the puppies on social media pages to see if I could see them - not really with the intention of buying one, just mainly to see how cute they were, at least that's what I told myself.

When I came across the advert for Cavoodle puppies in our hometown of Collie, I showed it to Rod. I really wanted a Cavoodle for our next dog and even though I thought the timing wasn't right, something in my soul knew better. I sent a text in response to the advert; I only signed my name as Christine and didn't give my last name. I went to bed thinking nothing more of it.

Saturday morning, I woke up to a phone call from the puppy breeder, asking if I was Christine Keep. I was surprised that she asked my surname. I said, "Yes that's me." She replied that she had a feeling it was me and that she had four male puppies left. She'd heard how much I love dogs and said she would be very happy if one of them came to me. I thought about that after and knew that the Universe had put us together.

Rod and I went to look at the pups, making no commitment other than to look. Once we got there, I knew we would be leaving with one. We chose Ben, who turned out to be the cheekiest of them all and within a space of an hour we were home with a new member of our family. When I look back on this now, I know why Ben had come into our lives at this moment. He was an amazing distraction for us when Rod's health took a turn for the worse.

December 2022

The December scan came around very quickly and after it was done, we continued packing the caravan, ready to head away on holiday. Rod, being a contract manager, was responsible for hosting his employees' Christmas party. This was scheduled for the night of December 16th, less than a week after the CT scan and only six days from our planned holiday.

We were getting ready to head to the Christmas party when the phone call came from the cardiologist. My heart missed a beat, as she was only going to ring if there was something they picked up on the scan. Rod put her on speaker phone so we could both listen, as she told him the scan had showed the dye wasn't getting through the right chamber of his heart. She said it could be a faulty scan or that the picture didn't show it accurately. It was most likely nothing to worry about, but she wanted him to have an internal ultrasound (TOE) to make sure. What alarmed me most was that she wanted it done before Christmas. If she wasn't concerned, then why the hurry?

The feeling I'd had back in July, the one that had taken hold in my soul, suddenly seemed so much larger and heavier and I felt like we about to board a runaway train. We were both confused, is it just a faulty scan? Could there be something wrong with his heart? Why such a hurry to get the scan done? We tried to push the fears to the back of our minds and put on brave faces that night at the Christmas party with his colleagues and staff. We spoke to our friends to let them know that we might be a little delayed getting away, depending on when the ultrasound was arranged for. We told a few friends at the party what was going on, and they were all very comforting and reassuring.

The next day we got the booking date for the ultrasound, the twenty-third of December, in the morning. We packed up and went to stay in Mandurah at Kate's house. It was her birthday on the twenty-first of December, and we were going out for dinner with family and her friends. It was a welcome relief, from the stress of waiting for the ultrasound. Although it was an anxious wait, we were happy spending time with family.

December 23, 2022 - We headed to the hospital for the internal ultrasound appointment. We were told it was a short procedure under light sedation, undertaken by a cardiology specialist. Rod was admitted and was settled into the ward in readiness. The cardiologist came to see us and told us he had looked at the CT scan; he also didn't feel there was anything to worry about and that this would just be a routine check to make sure. He said Rod would be in and out within the hour. Reassured by this, I gave Rod a kiss and told him I would head off to have a coffee in the hospital café and be back when he's awake.

As I sat in the hospital coffee shop garden, I felt this wave of heaviness wash over me. My heart was pounding, and I felt very anxious. I told myself I was tired and stressed and it would be okay. I thought I was picking up on the energy of the hospital with so many patients in there, something as an empath I was prone to. When I arrived back at the ward Rod was back from the procedure, awake, pale, and groggy. I bent to give him a kiss on the forehead and asked, "How did it go?"

What came out of his mouth left me reeling with shock. "Not good, they think I have a tumour." I immediately thought to myself *he must be confused, it's the anesthetic reacting with him, he must have misunderstood what they had told him.*

One of the nurses came in and I told her what he had said. The look on her face and the way she reached out to take my hand told me something was very wrong. She said, "I'll get the doctor to come and talk with you." My whole body stood frozen, I couldn't even get my words out, I just nodded at her and as she left, I sat down in the chair next to Rod's bed and just stared at him.

It was a short while later when the cardiologist came in. He explained that he had seen something on the ultrasound, it appeared that something was blocking the right chamber of Rod's heart, a mass of some sort and he was organizing an urgent CT scan and possibly an MRI. I was in shock. I kept looking at Rod in disbelief. There was some confusion at that time whether they were going to keep Rod in hospital or whether he could come home that night. I think everyone was thrown into chaos that morning with what they had seen on the ultrasound and were unsure how to proceed. I made a phone call to Kate and as I was trying to tell her, all I could do was cry. She kept asking, 'Mum, what's wrong' and when I finally managed to tell her, she told me she was coming straight away to the hospital. We decided not to call Michael and Melissa until we knew more. Rod didn't want to stress them, especially as Michael lives in Darwin in the Northern Territory, three hours flight away.

Kate rushed to the hospital to be with us and waited with us until the scans were arranged. They wheeled Rod off for what was to be one of the most important scans of his life, and we went to sit in the coffee shop garden while he was away, both crying, both of us fearful and still in shock. When he came back from the scan, they told us that they had only undertaken a CT scan, that they had enough information and didn't need to do the MRI. I found that unsettling - what does that mean, they had enough information? Could that be a good thing, or what had they seen was enough that they didn't need to do the MRI? The cardiologist said he would call us later that day, when he had the full report, but it was okay for Rod to go home. The Cardiologist was going on Christmas leave along with many others in the medical profession but assured us he would have some answers for us quickly. We initially went back to Kate's to talk more with her and Kev, but then decided to return to our home, one and a half hours away, so that we could begin to process what we had just been told and prepare for the news to come.

The trip home was the quietest, and felt like the longest drive ever. My mind was racing, lots of thoughts, disbelief, and shock. I was too scared to look at Rod in case he could read my mind, and I kept myself occupied with concentrating on driving. We made a few phone calls to family and told them once we knew what we were dealing with, we would call them again. When the call finally came at 6:00 p.m., two days before Christmas, we were told, "Rod you have a suspicious mass in your chest, 5-6 cm in size and possibly attached to your heart." He told us he was arranging more tests including a PET scan, an MRI and possibly a biopsy, and that he had referred us to another specialist who would take over from here. "They will be in touch after Christmas and try not to worry."

Try not to worry!!! They had just told my husband, two days before Christmas, that he had a suspicious mass. I wanted to scream but all I could do was cry. I was lightheaded and felt like my world was spinning out of control. It was like I was watching a movie in slow motion, seeing the characters on the screen, and not realizing they were us. I know this response is what we call in somatic therapy as disassociation, distancing myself from the actual reality of the trauma. It felt like I was outside of my body.

I looked at Rod in disbelief. This wasn't us; they must be talking about someone else; they've got it wrong. We looked at each other stunned, tears silently rolling down my cheeks. The reality setting in that my gorgeous husband has something seriously wrong with him.

To receive this news so close to Christmas was devastating. I had lost my father to mesothelioma on Christmas Day, and for me it felt like that nightmare was starting all over again. I remembered back to that time, the trauma of losing him, my grief and sadness. But this was far worse, this was my husband, the love of my life and the person I wanted to grow old with. Being Christmas, we knew that it would be unlikely we would get an appointment until the new year. It was going to be the longest wait ever.

I kept replaying the conversations over and over in my head. The scenes at the hospital, the phone call that night. It felt like my brain was in overload and I couldn't focus on anything else. I wasn't sleeping, just lying awake all night starting at Rod, pleading with the Universe to heal him. Bargaining that I would do anything if they could make him okay. I used to go outside and stare at the moon and the stars, crying and begging for help. Rod, on the other hand, was worried but kept telling me it's just a benign tumour it would be okay. Even back then his mindset and positive attitude to this news was amazing.

We cancelled our holiday away and tearfully started telling family and friends. The hardest phone calls to make were the ones to Rod's children, Michael & Melissa. My heart broke for them both. Melissa struggled so much through this period. I could hear the fear in her voice and the need for reassurance that her dad was going to be okay, which of course we couldn't give her. Michael is a bit like Rod, in so much as if he doesn't have to talk about it, it's not really happening. Even though, deep down I knew how scared he was. The support we received from everyone was amazing, but we pretty much went into seclusion, staying home on our own Christmas Day. Neither of us felt like celebrating Christmas. The antics of our new pup, Ben, and our older dog, Bodhi, kept us going through that period.

Those days between Christmas and New Year's I pretty much spent the whole time alternating between crying and journaling. I use my journal most days, it's how I process what is going on in my life and in my thoughts. If you were to read my journal from those days, it would seem like the ramblings of someone who had completely lost their mind. My thoughts were all over the place and I questioned everything. I questioned my spiritual beliefs, my faith in the medical system and my strength in myself to get through this. It was as though everything I believed in was no longer true. Every time the phone rang, we jumped, wondering if it was the specialist with news of the tests to come. We were desperately waiting to hear what the next steps would be.

We both knew we were headed for a rollercoaster ride with specialist consultations, scans, and more blood tests but we were completely unprepared for the emotional toll it would take. As a counsellor and somatic trauma therapist in private practice, I had just signed a lease with a colleague and friend, Jodi, to go into a new building. I tearfully told her that I wasn't going to be able to continue with the move. I felt so guilty at letting her down, letting my clients down. I cancelled some of my client appointments and referred others on. I felt at that moment I didn't have the emotional capacity to support myself, let alone others. My business went on hold as I prepared to support Rod through this.

January 2023

It was getting close to New Year's, and we decided we didn't want to stay home alone anymore. We went to stay with Kate, Kev and granddaughters, Layla and Hannah. We had decided not to tell the granddaughters anything until we knew what we were dealing with. Christmas and New Year's is supposed to be one of celebration, and holiday excitement and we didn't want to ruin this for them. We tried to put the worry out of our minds and spent those few days at the beach, playing cards in the evening and watching shows on TV that would distract our thoughts. With my thoughts often going to worst case scenario, I did wonder at times if this would be our last New Year's together, and my New Year's wish was to have my husband cured and well.

Rod was very calm; he always has such a positive mindset and was truly convinced this would be a benign tumour and nothing to worry about. Me, on the other hand and being highly intuitive, knew this was something far more serious. Whilst Rod managed to go on with life as best as he could, I fell into a big hole. Even with all my professional training, I felt useless when it came to supporting myself and him. I struggled to make sense of this, locked in my fear of *what if I lose him, how will I survive and what will become of me?* I started to isolate myself from everyone except Rod, Kate, Kev, and the girls.

Those days between Christmas into the first week of January seemed like the longest wait, but we knew that the specialist teams were working behind the scenes when we got the call to arrange a PET Scan and MRI. We also received the appointment to see the specialist, which was scheduled for January 6, 2023. When we arrived at the specialist appointment, he confirmed there were several tests required before a decision could be made about what to do, and likely a biopsy. He told us there was an entire team looking at this because it was an unusual case, being a tumour so close to the heart. He didn't feel it was attached to the heart, which was contrary to what the cardiologist who undertook the ultrasound had told us. He felt it was in the pericardial lining. My initial thoughts went to mesothelioma and when this specialist started asking about Rod's exposure to asbestos, I could see he was thinking the same.

The rest of January was spent with organising and attending scans, blood test after blood test and filling out paperwork. There was much confusion over the MRI, everyone telling us that it needed to be done in a hospital that had cardiac specialists. This was not a routine MRI. We were both very much overwhelmed by all of this, Rod was sometimes confused as to which test he was having at the time, which I recognize as a normal trauma response. We needed to write everything down carefully, as most of the scheduled appointments were at different hospitals and labs. As the navigator, I would get extremely frustrated with where to park and how to get there, and I started noticing if things weren't running smoothly, I would find myself melting down quickly.

Eventually we got a call from a cardiac thoracic surgeon, James, who had now taken over the case and scheduled us for a consultation. When we got to the appointment, he told us he had wanted to see Rod in person to assess his physical condition before deciding whether to perform the biopsy. His thoughts were that if Rod's physical health wasn't the best, and with the risks associated with a heart biopsy, it might have been ruled out. As we sat across the desk from him, I could see him observing us carefully, and I noticed he had the most intense eyes. It was like he was looking deeply into our souls, but I immediately felt calm and a sense of trust that we were with the right person. I also remember thinking his desk was way too tidy, there was nothing on it but a notepad, pen and his computer. He turned his computer screen around and showed us both the PET scan and MRI results, and explained it was, in fact, a primary tumour of the heart and all indications showed it was malignant and large but had not yet metastasized to anywhere else in his body and was not likely mesothelioma. When I asked what he thought it could be, he looked at me for quite a few moments, wondering whether in that moment how to answer me and choosing his words carefully. His response was, "It could be a number of things, and I am happy to go through those with you, however I'm not sure it would be helpful right at this moment. Would you like me to do this?" Rod and I looked at each other and we agreed that we would wait until we knew something more conclusive, even though we had both googled heart tumours extensively. As he continued to talk us through what would happen next, I sat there with tears rolling down my cheeks, wondering how could this amazing man with a heart of gold have cancer of the heart? It didn't make any sense.

Life was so unfair, and, in that moment, I thought all our hopes and dreams for the future seemed unattainable.

This wasn't our plan, we had so much we wanted to do with our lives, how could this be a part of it? We still didn't know what type of cancer we were dealing with. James looked between me and Rod, with tears rolling down my cheeks, he said to Rod, "Well at least you know she loves you." We all laughed at this. He confirmed that he was happy that Rod was physically healthy enough to do a biopsy, which would confirm what type of tumour this was. He was unsure which type of biopsy they would perform. He wanted to consult with his colleagues first and would let us know. His preference, at that stage, was an open chest biopsy where, if he got the opportunity, he could remove the whole tumour at the same time.

I had already been down the google rabbit hole and my fear was growing daily. I knew I had to do something to change my mindset if I was going to support Rod through this. I had to get my emotional strength back. This was going to be a long journey, and I didn't want to look back on this and wish I had done it differently.

February 2023

It took a short while for the biopsy appointment due to the rarity of this cancer. James was consulting with colleagues in America, as well as here in Australia. Collaboratively, they decided the best course of action was to perform a biopsy by inserting a tube through the vein in Rod's neck down to the heart, removing pieces of the tumour. This would be the least invasive procedure and pose the least risk to Rod. We got the call for the appointment on the first of February, at Hannah's birthday dinner.

We took that call outside of the restaurant, trying to hide from the grandchildren, and Kate came outside to find us as we discussed what the next steps would be. By now it was February, almost seven weeks since it was first discovered. It was hard not talking about it that night, celebrating Hannah's birthday, with this hanging over our heads. Layla, our other granddaughter, kept looking at me. She shares both mine and Kate's intuition and I could see that she knew something was going on, and without making a big deal of it, she kept giving my hand a squeeze and a gentle reassurance with her presence.

On the day of the biopsy, Rod was prepped for the procedure and James told us it would be another surgical cardiologist undertaking the biopsy, one that did these procedures routinely. James is a leading cardiothoracic surgeon in Perth and assured us that he and his team would in the room, ready to step in if things went wrong, at which point he would perform open heart surgery. He also told us the pathologist would be in the room to assess whether they had enough tissue to complete testing. We knew this procedure came with some risks and once again I was left to wait, with Kate by my side, while he went to theatre. All we wanted was to know what we were dealing with. James rang me a short while later to tell me that the procedure went well, they had collected some tissue to send off for testing, and were hopeful they could get a result within a week, I was relieved and looked forward to getting Rod home. Rod was released later that day with just a minor incision in his neck and had to take it easy for a few more days. He was still working from home, and we tried to go on as normal.

The waiting was awful. I could tell that this was starting to put a strain on Rod - every time his mobile phone rang, we would both look, each anxiously, in case it was James. We wanted to know what it was, but at the same time we didn't, because if it was malignant we knew that this journey was going to be very difficult. When the call finally came, we were left frustrated and emotional. James told us that they couldn't get a diagnosis because the pieces of the tumour they removed had already died and the other tissue collected was healthy heart tissue. This meant that now Rod had to go for full thoracic surgery to obtain a surgical biopsy, which came with more risks and a longer stay in hospital. We were devastated; this meant more waiting and another procedure for Rod. I thought to myself, *how much more does this man have to go through to just be told what it is we are dealing with?*

Here we were, nearly 10 weeks on, still unsure what this monster was that was growing in his chest and with no idea what the future held for us.

CHAPTER TWO: THE DIAGNOSIS

Rod's second biopsy was scheduled for February 23, 2023, at the Mount Hospital in Perth, Western Australia. We headed to the city the day before, spending the night at a hotel near the hospital, where I would also stay for the next few nights so that I could be close by. We spent a lovely afternoon and evening together, enjoying each other's company. We laughed, I cried, and we reminisced about some of the most memorable moments of our lives together. It was the most connected we had felt to each other in a long time. I also felt I was my most vulnerable with him.

We got back to the hotel room and Rod started his fast in preparation for the surgery, when James called him at 8:30 in the evening. We were used to James ringing us late, but hadn't been expecting a phone call from him that night. He told us that the Mount Hospital had an air-conditioning issue and they had cancelled all surgeries for the next day. His exact words were, *you couldn't make this stuff up if you tried*. He was so apologetic; he knew how desperate we were for answers. He told us he was trying to reschedule Rod's biopsy for one day later at another hospital, where he assured us, he often performed surgery. He indicated he would confirm if this was possible in the morning, and once again, the rollercoaster ride was in full swing.

The biopsy was confirmed for Friday at the St John of God Hospital Subiaco. Rod checked into the hospital early as requested, and, once again, I kissed him a tearful goodbye with the promise that I would be back when he was awake. I went back to the hotel for a short while to try and get some rest. Neither of us had slept much the night before and I was exhausted by the worry and constant changing of plans. By the time I got back to the hospital Rod had just returned to his room and was in a lot of pain. I hate seeing him in pain, especially as he isn't a person who normally shows it. It wasn't long before James came in to speak with us. He said the surgery had gone well; he'd had to make an incision between Rod's ribs and stretch the muscles apart which was the cause of his extreme pain. He had taken about ten samples of tissue and was confident that they would be able to make a diagnosis from those. A piece had been rushed to the pathologist to get the process started, but it still might take up to 10 days for a full diagnosis. The thought of waiting another two weeks was almost too much to bear.

With Rod in so much pain, heavily medicated and drifting in and out of sleep, I left him to rest and drove home to Kate's, wanting to be as close as I could to her and the girls. I felt guilty leaving him, even though there wasn't anything I could do as I knew the nurses would be in and out all night, doing their checks and managing his pain medication. I think guilt is the hardest emotion to cope with. The guilt and sense of hopelessness at not being able to fix this or help him was enormous. It was the first time we had been apart since learning of the tumour.

As the anesthetic was wearing off, Rod was calling me on and off during the late afternoon and into the early evening, forgetting that he had just called me half an hour earlier. This wasn't new to me, as he had done this through previous surgeries. It was something I used to tease him about as he had no idea that he was doing it. When he called again at 6:00 p.m., I had a little laugh to myself thinking *here we go again, about to have the same conversation over*. But this time was different, he sounded more alert and told me that James had been back in to see him and that they had a preliminary diagnosis - angiosarcoma. As soon as the words came out of his mouth my head started spinning and I sat back on the bed, frightened I was about to pass out. Once again, I went into silent movie mode, feeling like I had left my body. Rod told me that James had already been speaking with an oncologist some days prior, as they had already suspected what this was. Rod told me that both James and the oncologist wanted to meet with us both tomorrow morning at the hospital to discuss what would happen from here. I tearfully said goodbye to him, hoping he would finally get some sleep.

As I walked into the kitchen to tell Kate, she could see something was horribly wrong. I saw the colour drain from her face as she ushered me back into the bedroom where we could talk. It was our worst nightmare. Primary cardiac angiosarcoma, an extremely rare and aggressive cancer with a very poor prognosis. When we look at the statistics at the time of writing this book there is only one in 36 million diagnosed with this cancer. We were both in shock.

Again, we decided not to tell the granddaughters until after the meeting the next day, but it was becoming increasingly difficult to hide my fear and pain from them. Layla, the oldest granddaughter, was noticing something was wrong, asking me why I was crying. I had no words to say to her other than we'd had some bad news, and I was very sad. We didn't elaborate, but deep down I think both the girls knew this was to do with grandpa and that he was very sick.

I knew I had to let Rod's brothers know about the diagnosis. As I mentioned, they are a very tight knit family, and Rod and I often joke that when you marry into the Keep family, you have to have the approval of the brothers. Ken was in Thailand getting married and I tried to get hold of him but I couldn't, so I left a message to ring me. My next call was to Gary, and as I tearfully told him of the news I could tell he was shocked and didn't know what to say. He asked if I had got hold of Ken. Ken is considered the patriarch in their family, being the eldest, and he's the one the brothers confer to in family emergencies. I explained I had tried and would keep trying, and he offered to also try. My next call was to Shane, and at this point I was done holding it all together; when he answered I told him through my sobs. He was devastated and tried to be supportive, but I could hear the fear in his voice. The video call came from Ken, not long after, and I quickly knew that Gary or Shane had already spoken with him. At this point, I was completely out of control and as much as I was trying to be strong, I broke down completely. Ken wanted to come home immediately but I told him that Rod would not want that. We all wanted him to marry Kai, and to welcome her into the Keep family. This was far too important, and I assured him there wasn't much he could do at this point and we could continue to keep him informed as we knew more.

I didn't sleep much that night, all these thoughts rolling around in my head. I spent the night crying, snoozing, waking and crying again, trying not to let anyone else in the house hear me. Picturing Rod all alone in the hospital bed, having been told he has one of the most aggressive and rare cancers a person could possibly have. My thoughts were all about the future and the uncertainty of what the specialists wanted to talk to us about. What if they told us there was nothing more could be done? What if they told me that Rod was going to die. The pain that night was almost too much to bear.

The next morning, with red and bleary eyes and a massive headache from lack of sleep, I walked into the hospital with Kate by my side. Rod was still in a lot of pain, and I could see he was worn out. He kept pressing the button to give himself more pain relief and was anxiously watching for the green light so he could press it again. I found this hard to watch. We met with James first, who confirmed they had suspected it was this all along, and that he had managed to get a good look at the tumour whilst doing the biopsy. He told us it was too large and too dangerous at this stage to try and remove it. It would do too much damage to Rod's heart, and he might not survive the surgery. This was a blow to Rod, who had his hopes set that they would be able to remove it and then have further treatment. He told us that he had arranged for Associate Professor, Dr. Tim Clay (Medical Oncologist) to come and meet with us. The reason he had spoken to Tim was because this was such a rare cancer with not many cases in Australia, and Tim had treated a patient before with this diagnosis.

It was the early afternoon when Tim came to see us. He asked Rod a few questions about his lifestyle and our family, and generally spent time getting to know him. He told us the plan would be to try to shrink the tumour with chemotherapy, with a view to removing it surgically later. He said his goal would be to get Rod into remission. He spoke about how the chemotherapy would mean Rod would lose all his hair and had other side effects which he would go into when we next met with him. Tim also asked us if we would like to be part of a research program where they could look for targeted treatment, and because this was such a rare cancer, we wouldn't have to pay for it. We both agreed to this, whatever information they could gain from this might not only help Rod but others as well. We instantly felt in good hands with him, and it was in this moment that we knew Tim was going to be a big part of our lives.

Kate and I spoke about how relieved we were that they had a plan and hadn't just told us there was nothing more they could do. Rod was staying in for another night, and I told Kate I would stay with him for the afternoon, and it was okay for her to go home. She was exhausted herself from these last few weeks and trying to be strong for us, and I knew she needed to be with her husband and the girls.

As I was walking Kate out, I knew I had to make the phone calls to Michael and Melissa. I left a message for Mel but got hold of Michael. I held back my tears as I told him the diagnosis and the plan going forward. I begged him not to google it because what he would read was terrifying. I explained that the information on google is out of date because this is a rare cancer and there aren't many case studies. When Mel rang back later that day, I knew she had already spoken with Michael. She was scared, tearful and terrified of losing her dad. I reassured her that right now he was okay and that when they released him tomorrow, he would call her. I knew that both had already googled cardiac angiosarcoma and read that the life expectancy without surgical removal was only 7-12 months, with no cure, so I completely understood their fears. As a counsellor I know that the brain has a way of distorting an image and that you need to see the person to reassure yourself that they are okay in that moment. I promised Mel she would be able to see him soon. I realized later, that when we were talking with Tim I had forgotten to ask about the long-term prognosis, or what the outcome had been for his one other patient with this type of cancer. On reflection, even if I had, I know he would not have been able to answer me.

When I look back to this time, telling Rod's children and his brothers were some of the hardest calls I had ever had to make. Telling my family and friends seemed easier, partly because they know me so well and I could be my authentic, vulnerable self with them, whereas with Rod's family, I felt I had to be stronger and more in control.

James kept checking in on Rod, between his surgeries throughout that day, and at one when point with Rod was in the bathroom, he asked me how I was dealing with this. I started to cry, admitting I was very scared. He put his hand on my arm to comfort me and one of the nurses put her arms around my shoulders. I knew that what we were dealing with was extremely serious, and with not much known about this cancer it must have been hard for them to watch our fear. At this stage, James was confident that if Tim could shrink the tumour, Rod may still be able to have surgery to remove it and he assured us he would be monitoring Rod's progress carefully.

On my way back to Kate's that evening, she rang to say it was time to tell the granddaughters. We no longer wanted to hide the truth from them. Although we would still censor how much information to give them, Kev and Kate decided they would tell them grandpa was sick and would have to have treatment, but stop short of telling them it was cancer. If we used the word *cancer*, Layla would have googled it, and we didn't need them to worry or be sad any more than necessary. When I got home, we gathered together and explained about all the tests and the surgery, and that grandpa needed treatment. Layla asked if that was why grandpa had been in Perth for lots of appointments, and why we had been staying with them so much. When we told her yes, she replied, "So, that's why you look like you're about to cry all the time Nanna." You can't hide much from children; I find they are silent observers. We explained that we hadn't told them earlier as we hadn't wanted to worry them. We explained that this treatment would be hard on him, and he might feel nauseous, and was going to lose his hair. Rod has thick hair and Hannah, the youngest, often calls him her hairy monkey. When we told them about the hair, Hannah cried out. "Noooo, not Grandpa's soft hair." They asked when he was coming home, which was probably the following day, to which Hannah asked, "Will his hair be all gone by then?" This made us laugh. I told her we would probably shave his hair off which would be easier than watching it fall out. Layla thought it would be a great idea to give him a mohawk first. For a few moments we could laugh at their innocence, and it took our minds off the current reality.

Kate and Kev had made plans the previous September to buy a caravan, sell their home, quit their jobs, home school the girls and travel Australia for a year. They were set to leave in April, only two months away. This decision was now weighing heavily on their minds, knowing how serious Rod's condition was and the uncertain future ahead of us. They were torn between wanting to continue with their dreams, yet wanting to spend as much quality time with Rod as possible and be there to support me. Kate said she didn't want to leave me to deal with this alone. We talked it over several times and both Rod and I told them to continue with their dream of travelling. If we needed them, they were only a plane flight away and part of me wanted to shelter Kate and the granddaughters from what was to come. One thing we have learnt from this is not to put dreams on hold, because life can change in a moment.

Rod came home from hospital the next day, still in a lot of pain and it took him the next two weeks to recover from the surgery. Tim rang to let us know that he wanted to see us on the 15th of March, and that treatment would begin that day, however he wanted another PET scan so he could see the size of the tumour as a benchmark before treatment commenced. By this time, it was nearly three months since the tumour had been discovered and my fear was that it had grown and spread to other areas of the body. Once again, I went down the google rabbit hole, consumed by my research. The hours I spent on the internet left me exhausted and the more I read, the more depressed I became. I hid a lot from Rod, but little did I know he was doing the same thing.

I felt like I wanted to know everything about chemotherapy, what to expect, and was fearful of how he would cope. I wanted to build his immune system up as much as possible and began researching diets, lifestyle changes and much more to give him the best outcome when dealing with the treatment.

We headed to Perth where Rod would have the PET scan on March 14th. Rod had to fast for 16 hours and by the time the scan was over he was very hungry. We went to lunch and tried to calm our nerves about what to expect the next day. The following morning, we headed into Tim's office, prepared as best we could for chemo but nervous for what he might say. As we sat in his office, he delivered the bombshell news. The tumour had grown significantly in size and had spread to both his lungs. This had been our biggest fear since learning of the diagnosis, and the frustration of waiting so long. He confirmed this was now classified as 'advanced cancer' and we would be treating it aggressively. He explained that it had the jump on Rod, and we had a lot of ground to make up. Chemotherapy would begin weekly for twelve weeks using a drug called Paclitaxel, with another drug called Doxorubicin - the Red Devil - being added every three weeks. He would be starting both drugs that day. We now know why they call the drug Doxorubicin the Red Devil.

It was going to be a long and hard road ahead.

CHAPTER THREE: THE TREATMENT BEGINS

We left Tim's rooms and headed downstairs to the chemotherapy suite, known as the Ivy Suite, in the Bendat Cancer Centre, Subiaco, Western Australia. This was going to be our new norm for the next three months; a quick appointment in Tim's office to review Rod's weekly blood tests and assess his side effects, then head to the chemo suite. We were quiet on the way there, both in shock over the news it had spread, almost doubled in size, and scared about chemotherapy. No one can prepare you for the overwhelm that cancer brings, let alone the fears over the treatment.

Whilst Rod was in the toilet prior to entering the Ivy Suite, I rang Kate to tell her this new news and desperately trying not to cry. With only a few minutes to talk, I told her that we had spoken extensively to Tim, and what the treatment consisted of. I was scared and I could tell that this new information was playing heavily on their minds too, especially as they were leaving the next month. We headed into the chemotherapy suite, fearful and sad.

Some people elect not to undergo chemo, instead trying natural therapies first. These thoughts had crossed my mind as well, especially as I'm very much about energy therapy and the ability of our bodies to heal themselves. I personally believe that most illnesses and diseases are a result of either an emotional, physical or environmental imbalance. Please know that I am in no way advocating that you disregard recommendations from the medical profession when treating diseases such as these, and I encourage everyone to use all the information presented to them to make an informed decision. In this case, we knew that Rod's best chance of survival, or at least to prolong his life, was to have the chemotherapy and we put our trust in Tim to provide the best medical care and options available. I would be able to support his body with complimentary therapies such as breathwork, sound meditation and reiki for relaxation, as we progressed.

We were told there was to be an education session on the treatment; what to expect; what to look out for; who to ring in an emergency and a whole lot more information to digest. This would mean we would be in the chemo suite for most of the day. When I think back to that day now, I realise how unprepared we were. Rod was putting on a brave face and as he sat in the chair to start his treatment, my heart broke again. He looked so small in the chair and so scared, even though he was trying hard not to show it. I kept asking myself why this was happening to him. I was struggling to hold it all together and excused myself to go to the toilet so I could cry.

The nurses always seem to have difficulty getting a canula into Rod's veins, and today was no different. It took four nurses and six attempts before they could start the treatment. I could see the pain on Rod's face, but he bravely sat there and tried to smile through it. I managed to get Rod doing some deep breaths to help relax his muscles and his veins, and we both breathed a sigh of relief when they finally got the needle in. I hoped that it wouldn't be like this each week.

Rod was given pre-meds, and then the first chemotherapy drug, Doxorubicin - the Red Devil - was administered through an injection directly into the vein. So far, so good, no adverse reactions. After a short break, the next drug, Paclitaxel, was administered through the IV line.

We saw so many people on that first day, and with so much information it was a lot to take in. I wrote lots of notes so that I would remember everything. The nurses in the chemo suite were incredible. They recognized how anxious we were and tried to make the process as easy as possible. We had small banter, a few laughs, and a joke at Rod's expense with me telling him they were "marinating him"... something we often joke about now, referring to it as marinating day.

When I looked around the suite, I saw so many people coming and going. As soon as one chair was empty, it was cleaned, and another patient arrived. This went on all day. It was a shock to see just how many people's lives are affected by cancer. We read about it, see it on the news, hear of friends having a cancer diagnosis, but nothing is like the harsh reality you see in the chemo suite. This is only one chemo suite of the hundreds all over Australia alone. It was mind blowing and so sad to think that so many were going through what we were.

Five hours after it began, it was over. The first treatment day was behind us. We headed home with a chemo pack full of information, anti-nausea drugs and steroids. Unsure of what to expect with the side effects we had been told may occur, I had already prepared for the long drive home. I had sick bags, wipes, a towel, and water in the car. What I didn't realise was that with the pre-meds he was given, Rod probably wouldn't start to feel the side effects until the next day or longer.

I kept asking him how he was feeling over and over. It must have frustrated him, but I was expecting him to be worse than he was. I realised, for us it was nothing like you see in the movies. Each person's chemo experience is different. What we've learnt through this is that everyone reacts differently to the treatment and needs to find their own mindset to approach the process with a positive attitude. Rod was having two of the strongest drugs and we were lucky that nausea wasn't an issue with him. To date he has not had to take any of the nausea medication aside from the steroids in the first few days following the Doxorubicin treatments.

We slipped quickly into the routine of chemotherapy. It seemed like we lived our lives in terms of the days leading up to chemo or days after. Having weekly chemo, meant that Rod also had to have a weekly blood test the day before treatment, and on the day of treatment he would see either Tim or his oncology nurse, Kate. He became a human pin cushion. We had talked to the nurses about putting in a port to make the insertion of the needle easier, but because of the risk to the heart this was ruled out which meant a canula in his arm or hand each week. I was so proud of the way Rod handled this. Some weeks they got the line in on the first attempt, others it took several tries. I found myself getting nervous each time, and after getting him to do some deep breathing I would have to walk away so that I couldn't see his pain.

After the first few weeks we became old hands, and we could tell who all the newbies were that came into the suite. They all looked like we had that first day - scared, not smiling, still in shock, nervously glancing at everyone else, worried family and friends by their side supporting them. It sounds wrong to say we were old hands by now, I even remember talking to Kate about Rod's chemo bag filled with all the things to make him more comfortable during the treatment. Who the hell has a chemo bag? How awful does that sound? Yet, the sad reality is many people have a chemo bag and I often wonder how many bags are purchased just to take to chemotherapy.

I love to write; I sometimes write poetry, other times just reflections that I share with my journal. Writing helps me to make sense of my reality and helps me find the words to support others - it helps me to be authentically me. I would reflect on the chemo suite often and I wrote this one day whilst sitting waiting for Rod to have treatment.

> I look across the room at others in the chemo suite,
> some of them alone, some with family & friends.
> Each with a different story, a different cancer,
> and a different diagnosis.
>
> Yet here we are all sitting in the same place,
> fearful but putting on a brave face and I meet their
> eyes with a soft smile and an inner knowing that says,
> "I see you".
>
> Some don't want to look around. They come with their
> loved ones with their eyes cast down. Still in disbelief
> that this is now their life. They sit and support the one
> hooked up to the special drug, hopeful that it works,
> silently locked in their own grief.
>
> The nurses are busy, so many to see. Short-staffed and
> hungry but not taking a break even as they bring us
> cups of tea. Their joyful smiles and cheerful jibes are a
> welcome relief from the fear, sadness, and disbelief.
>
> They, and the others make it more bearable, and as
> our turn comes to an end for today, we smile and say
> thank you and turn and walk away.
>
> Knowing we will be back next week with another
> room full of strangers to greet.

Rod's side effects were getting worse each week. He had gastrointestinal issues, a horrific full body rash, sore nails and feet and had lost most of the hair on his body by week three. I was paranoid about him catching something, with his immune system dropping each week. The morning after a treatment, and it appeared to be more when he had the Doxorubicin, he would develop this weird hiccup. It would occur at random times of the day and only one hiccup. Then, just as quickly as it appeared, it was gone. It only occurred for the first day after treatment. I'm not sure if it's the steroids they give him or the treatment itself. The first couple of nights after treatment he would find it very hard to sleep, another effect of the steroids, and we would try to keep him awake as long as possible, hoping he was so tired he would manage to sleep. We found that it was important for Rod to rest during the day, usually in the afternoon and just for an hour or so. This helped him recover between treatments more quickly, and he balanced this with pottering around in his shed and doing light exercise.

We still had Covid hanging around our hometown, and I asked our visitors to wear a mask. I went into overdrive with cleaning and disinfecting every time anyone came over, almost becoming obsessive, and it wasn't long before I was both physically and emotionally exhausted.

Both Rod and I are well known in town, so every time I went to the supermarket I would run into someone we knew. It felt like I was repeating the same trauma over and over. Each time I knew I had to go there I got more and more stressed. I was wearing a mask and constantly sanitizing everything, just like we did back in the early days of Covid. I kept my eyes down and tried to avoid people. Eventually I started online grocery shopping as a way of avoiding people and potential germs or viruses, but this only isolated me further.

We were prisoners in our own home. Not only had the cancer robbed us of our future hopes and dreams, but now it was robbing us of any small happiness we had in this moment. By week six we were both exhausted. Each Wednesday was chemo day, and we would leave home at 6:30 a.m., drive 200 km to get to the cancer hospital, spend most of the day there and return home about 6:00 p.m. I found myself spending the next day on the couch, emotionally and physically spent. As time went on, I noticed it was taking me longer to get dressed in the morning. Often sitting in my dressing gown until 10:00 a.m. The dogs weren't getting walked and everything was slipping behind. I knew that, once again, something had to change.

Rod has always been a social person, involved over the years in various sports and clubs. Working in the power station, he had a large team of colleagues, and I could see he was starting to miss the social interaction with others. It was hard watching him like this, but the fear of him catching something weighed heavily on me. I was trying to control the outcome and I felt guilty and frustrated at the same time. I just wanted to get to the end of the treatment, promising myself it would be better then.

Rod's next PET scan was due for week 10 of the treatment cycle, once again scheduled the day before the Tim's appointment and treatment. I remember being extremely nervous about this one. What if the treatment wasn't working, what if it had spread? These thoughts kept playing over and over in my mind. I was praying that the tumour had shrunk, putting that intention out into the universe. Rod was simply hoping it had shrunk enough for him to have surgery.

We nervously sat in Tim's room waiting to be called in. The moment arrived, and when he put the two scans on the screen, the one prior to treatment and the one taken yesterday, we held our collective breath. I could hear my heart pounding in my chest and my eyes were locked intently on him, as he told us, "The tumour has shrunk, as have the spots in your lungs, and at this point it has been put to sleep."

I was confused and asked, "What does this mean, put to sleep?"

He responded by saying, "I don't want you to rush out of here thinking it's gone, but at this moment it's not currently active, which is the best outcome we could have asked for."

I started to cry; it was asleep. My husband wasn't going to die within the time frame I had read on google. I felt such a release in that moment as I realised just how much I had been holding onto my emotions, pushing through week after week. Tim told us that the problem they face now is with this cancer being so rare, there is no real protocol for treating it. He had hit it hard and Rod's body was still doing okay, but the next hurdle was deciding what to do next. We knew we still had three more treatments until the end of the three-month cycle and Tim assured us he would have a plan for going forward. He needed to consult with the sarcoma team and let us know what the options would be. It was a small win and it felt like all the isolation and exhaustion was worth it now.

Rod's immune system was holding its own. The chemotherapy side effects, while sometimes debilitating and uncomfortable, were manageable. This was the first glimmer of hope in a long time. Our goal was to get Rod to surgery where we could get this monster in his chest removed. We also decided we'd had enough of living in isolation and fear, being too scared to go out, too scared to see people, too scared of Rod catching something. We were going to get on with living.

I started going downtown a bit more often, still wearing my mask. I had not been to a hairdresser for about six months, mainly because I was consumed with supporting Rod. I booked an appointment and for the first time whilst I was out, I took off my mask at the hairdresser's. I noticed a woman next to me had come in wearing a mask and was coughing, even though she reassured everyone she didn't have Covid. I was uneasy and my intuition radar was on high alert. As soon as I could put a mask back on, I did, but it was too late. Within a couple of days of that appointment I had Covid. In the three years that Covid had been around, neither Rod nor I had caught it. I was devastated and angry at myself, guilty that it was me who put him at risk. Rod had a few friends offer to drive him to chemo and we took advantage of this. As if cancer wasn't isolating enough, now I had to isolate from Rod. I was very ill from Covid and very emotional, and I spent most of those ten days crying, sleeping, in pain and hardly eating. I had a quick trip to the hospital because of the chest and back pain I was experiencing with Covid and asked a friend drive me. It turned out that the Covid infection was being unkind to my kidneys. I have polycystic kidney disease and the doctor at the hospital thought that Covid was responsible for this pain. My kidney function had dropped. This was hard for Rod because he couldn't do anything for me and we were so used to being together, supporting each other, but there was no way I could risk his life. Eventually, after two weeks I tested negative, although it was a few more weeks before I was completely recovered and we got back on track.

We made it to the final treatment day, when Tim delivered us another blow. The sarcoma team wanted to take a "watch and wait" approach. Surgery was out of the question because the cancer had already metastasized to his lungs. Tim felt a watch and wait with angiosarcoma was far too risky and wanted to keep going with maintenance chemo; he would talk further with a colleague about the plan going forward. The rug had been pulled out from underneath us again.

Tim told us that Rod needed at least a one week break following his final treatment, to rest and recover. He said that he had pushed Rod hard and was pleased he hadn't put him in hospital with the treatment. He would have a few options for us to consider within a week's time.

That night, as we sat and reflected on the day, I could see that Rod was devastated. He turned to me and questioned what had been the point of being so strong these three months of treatment, if they aren't going to remove it. I was crushed to see him like this. I told him the point of being strong was that both he and Tim had put it to sleep. I reassured him how much his own mindset and body had played a huge part in this, as had Tim's treatment plan.

Whilst I was sad for Rod, I was relieved that we had come to the end of this aggressive treatment. His fingernails and toenails had all gone black and were lifting, his nose and eyes were watering constantly and his body was physically exhausted. He needed this break... we needed this break. But Rod being Rod, didn't take long to regain his positive mindset and we waited for the options going forward.

A week's break turned into two. Tim had spoken to us over the phone about Rod's options which he then put into an email for us to consider.

Option 1 - A watch and wait approach to see what the tumour does for the next three months.

Option 2 - Continue with Paclitaxel on a three week on and one week off cycle.

Option 3 - Change to a new drug, Caelyx, a form of Doxorubicin but less damaging to the heart, to be administered every four weeks.

We went back with several questions to help us make an informed decision as this was left up to us to decide. Up to this point we had still not discussed Rod's long-term prognosis. I wanted to know if even with maintenance chemo would the cancer eventually become resistant, or if we decided to go with watch and wait and it wakes up, will he be back on the same aggressive treatment as before? We also wanted to know if surgery may be considered as an option in the future. I threw in a cheeky question, "If this was you, Tim, which option would you choose?".

While we waited for Tim's response, Rod and I tried to talk through the options presented to us. Rod takes a little while to process things and I was frustrated that he couldn't seem to decide. As a counsellor, I understand how important it is for the person to feel like they have a voice and control over their treatment plan, but when it came to Rod, I was wishing someone could just make the decision for us. It felt as though whichever option we chose there were risks involved.

When the email response finally came, I noticed that Tim had sent it at midnight on a Sunday. It made me reflect on what his life must be like and how much he must care about his patients, as well as trying to balance his own personal life. It was a detailed response which, once again, left me reeling. He intimated that this cancer was not going to stay away, it would eventually wake up and when it did, he would like to get another biopsy for genomic testing to see if there was a targeted treatment we could use. When they did the initial biopsy, they had used all the tissue to make a diagnosis so unfortunately genomic testing at that point wasn't possible. Tim also confirmed in his reply, that to prolong Rod's life and give him the best quality of life, he would suggest not taking the watch and wait approach. He felt that this was far too risky. If it was him in Rod's position, he would take option three, the monthly treatment with the new drug. He also confirmed that there was a possibility that the cancer may become resistant to chemotherapy.

This was the first time we fully understood that Rod would never be completely cured. If he stopped chemo, the chances were that the cancer would wake up quickly. Our best hope was to try and keep it asleep for as long as possible. After a couple of sleepless nights and lots of discussion, we decided to take option three. Having the chemo monthly meant that Rod could have some balance between treatment and lifestyle. Rod was still working from home, however he had a lot of personal leave owing and I suggested that now was the time to start taking it. This would give us the opportunity to take short trips away with our caravan in between treatment cycles.

It seemed a bit surreal at first, knowing the cancer was sleeping, with no idea for how long. We were convinced Rod was going to be the one who could beat this. He and Tim were going to keep it asleep, and we were going to get part of our lives back. I started to loosen my grip on wanting to control everything. It's a hard balance between wanting to protect him and trying to live a normal life, even though our lives felt anything but normal. For those past three months our whole focus had been on weekly chemo, and now we had four weeks to fill in between treatments. It was going to take some adjusting to. We made the decision right then, to live each day completely in the moment, making the most of the time we had together because no one could tell us how long that would be.

Our new normal was now monthly treatments, with three monthly PET scans to check what the cancer was doing. The PET scans always bring scanxiety in the week leading up to them. Rod can't consume carbohydrates within the 24 hours prior to the scan, and he starts the fasting process 16 hours prior. We often stay at the one of the Cancer Council lodges in Perth. There are two of them and they are available to anyone from Australia having cancer treatment or related appointments. This is such a gift to the community. On the day of the scan, I drop Rod off to the radiology department where he has radioactive dye injected into his body, and a full body scan to see what the cancer is doing and whether it has shown up anywhere else in his body. The whole process takes about three hours, and during that time, I wait in the nearby coffee shop, often writing in my journal.

We then have a nervous wait until we see Tim, either the next day or the day following, and we try to put the results out of our minds. Each scan we get, and Tim tells us the cancer is stable and still asleep feels, like a gift from the Universe. We can breathe a sigh of relief for the next three months.

It was also at this point we decided to take a trip away, giving Rod's body time to rest and recover in between treatments. We took our first trip to Shark Bay, some 800 km north of Perth, and spent a wonderful three weeks there with our friends, Matt and Kay, and their two children, Noah and Indi. Collie is cold in the winter and most houses have wood fires. This means lots of wood smoke in the air and I felt that we needed a break from this. It was hard enough for Rod having this cancer, we didn't need lung disease added to the mix.

I also decided that, with the future still unknown, I would not return to my business as it was before. Instead, I would start to document our journey through a social media blog with the aim of helping others feel less alone and confused as we were, and to give others hope for the future.

CHAPTER FOUR: THE HOLIDAY ODYSSEY

In September 2023 we started talking to Tim about the possibility of travelling to the eastern states of Australia for three months. We wanted to leave after the November scan and treatment, and hoped to meet up with Kate, Kev and the girls. Kate was turning 40 on December 21st, and we wanted to spend her birthday, then Christmas and January with them, hoping to make as many memories as we could. It was important for me that our granddaughters, Layla and Hannah, would look back on the time that we had travelled together as some of the fondest childhood memories. I was missing them desperately and felt such a strong urge to be with them.

I thought that if we gave Tim as much notice as possible it would be easier for him to make the arrangements. I had heard that others had managed to travel while having chemotherapy, and I was hoping that this would be the same for Rod. When we first approached the subject, we did so gently and I asked, "We were wondering if it's possible to travel for three months and have treatment in different states?" I explained what our plans were and the reasons why. I could see the look on his face, that look of 'oh my gawd'.

He quickly recovered his composure and said, "Yes, it is possible, a lot of stuffing around, but possible." My heart started to flutter, those words *it is possible* were all I heard. Our dreams of travelling further than our recent small trips were actually possible. I was elated. I was going to see my girls, I needed to see my girls.

Tim asked me to send an email outlining the dates we wanted to be away, and a rough plan of where we wanted to be for each chemo treatment. He also stipulated that it would hinge on Rod's next PET scan, due in November, with the proviso that if Rod started feeling unwell or any new symptoms appeared we would return home immediately. We agreed to this and went home to start the planning.

I was mapping out dates and places trying to determine where we would meet up with Kate and the family. We agreed that the best place and date to give us both time to get there would be December 16th in Eden NSW, where we would celebrate her birthday some five days later. For Rod and myself, this meant we both had something exciting to look forward to. Travelling Australia was our retirement dream. Even though we weren't retired and the travelling whilst having treatment looked a little different than our original vision, it was still a tick on the bucket list we had.

I sent Tim our itinerary, letting him know that we would fit in with the other treatment centres that he could refer us to and be happy to work around their schedules. We were so grateful just to be able to travel. We also let him know that we needed to be in NSW for December 16th. We had worked out that with Rod having chemo every four weeks, it meant that he would need three treatments while we were away and would have us back in time for his February PET scan. Tim sent off referrals to his colleagues in the East. We were hoping to have the first treatment in Port Pirie, South Australia, with the middle one in Victoria, possibly Traralgon, and the final one back in Port Pirie on the way home.

I could now understand why Tim had given me the look he had when I first mentioned it. Whilst the South Australian treatment was approved and seemed to be no problem, the Victorian one was proving more difficult. The Traralgon treatment centre wanted Rod to meet with the oncologist at least a week before his actual treatment day, as he was a new client. I tried to explain that we would still be in another state, NSW, at that point, and that we were only travelling so wouldn't need a second treatment there. I asked if he could do a video consult, which he declined, advising me he had to see the oncologist in person. I found that totally frustrating because all through the Covid pandemic in Australia, video appointments were second nature. There was no negotiating around this, and I tearfully ended the conversation with, "We will have to get back to you."

When we told Tim, his reaction was, "Well, that's a bit sad," and he asked us if we were prepared to go to Melbourne to St. Vincent's Private Hospital, where he had undertaken some training, as he would be able to make those arrangements. The email was sent off and it wasn't long before that appointment was confirmed, our plans were back on track, and we felt much more comfortable. Prior to Rod's diagnosis, something like this wouldn't have bothered me and I would have been able to cope, but after these long months, it was becoming very easy to unbalance and overwhelm me.

By October we were full steam ahead with packing and planning, but at the back of our minds was the upcoming PET scan. Our trip away hinged on a stable scan and getting the green light to go. As the scan drew closer, I became very agitated. I was longing to see Kate and had such high hopes that I was unsure how I would react if Tim told us we couldn't go. With this constantly on my mind, I left packing the essentials into our caravan until the very last minute. Normally Rod's PET scan appointments are scheduled on a Tuesday, the day before his oncology review and subsequent treatment. We found this to be the best option for us, as we never had to wait long for the results, which is something I hear that other people often do. However, this one in November was scheduled for the week before treatment and two weeks out from us leaving on our holiday.

Our mindsets focused on thinking positive thoughts. It's going to be okay. We will be going; we will continue manifesting this. Feathers started appearing every day and I would find them in random places. We were still experiencing rain, and rainbows were shining down outside my lounge window regularly. I took these as positive signs from the Universe. Yet there was still that slight fear of what if it's woken up? Our trip would be cancelled, and my heart completely shattered.

Rod's PET scan went ahead as scheduled and we held our breath, with a week to wait for the results seeming like an eternity. I stopped packing, telling myself that would be easier, if Tim gave us a red light instead of a green one. By the end of that week and only three days after the scan, my anxiety levels were through the roof. I suggested to Rod that maybe we could email Tim's admin, Gemma, to see if he can call us with the results. We agreed that we would.

I sent the email to Gemma, explaining that we didn't want to keep packing and thinking we were still leaving the day after treatment, because if the results were bad we would then have to unpack the caravan. I asked if it was possible, and Tim had time, we would appreciate if he could give us an indication before our appointment next week.

While we waited for a response, I kept looking at the weather forecast for our trip across the Nullabor. The Nullabor is what we call the stretch of road that connects Western Australia to South Australia, and is approximately 1200 km long. This stretch would be the longest we would have to drive in the shortest amount of time. We had hoped to be across it in two days. Now this might not seem such a big deal to some, but Rod, towing a caravan whilst having chemo treatment, meant it was going to be a tiring journey. He wasn't that keen on me driving, not that I know why. I consider myself to be a good driver and have towed trailers and horse floats, but not a caravan before. The weather on the way over wasn't going to be our friend and we were expecting 60 km side winds the whole way, which would make for an uncomfortable drive.

When Tim's oncology nurse, Kate, phoned on the Friday afternoon, I held my breath. Rod had taken the call outside and when he came back in, I nearly passed out when he told me, "It's stable and we can keep packing." She had told him the results were good and they would go through it in detail on Wednesday. I ran to him, sobbing with relief, and fell into his arms with a big hug. The cancer was still stable, Rod was doing okay, I would see my girls for the first time in eight months and our dreams were coming true.

After I managed to get some of my composure back, I immediately rang Kate and Kev. I knew they were anxiously awaiting the news themselves. It had been a tough year for us all and I think they wanted to see us as much as we did them. I video called her and played a bit of a trick, which was a little unfair. I said to her, "There's good and bad news. I will give you the bad news first." I saw the colour drain from her face so I quickly told her the weather was going to be awful on the Nullabor, but the good news was that we would be on it, and we would see them in a month's time. She dissolved into tears when the reality hit. We were coming. She went to Kev like I was with Rod, sobbing in his arms. I realised in this moment just how much stress they had been under this year as well, in coping with Rod's diagnosis. Even though they were on a trip of a lifetime, it weighed heavily on them that they were away from family and friends.

With this fabulous news, we went into overdrive packing. We had a week before departure day. It seemed a bit surreal, we would be leaving the safety and security of our home for a three-month trip away. Whilst this was a bucket list item for us, I was also slightly nervous about being so far away. But we had three months before the next scan, and we planned to make the most of that time, as best as we could. Rod loves fishing, so we loaded his boat on the roof of our Chevrolet truck, with him looking forward to spending time on the water at the various places we were headed to. He still had one more treatment to get through before departure day.

There were several people who helped us to make this trip a reality. We had needed some work done to our new Chevrolet Truck - in Australia we call it a Ute - to upgrade the suspension. Additionally, we wanted an annex fitted to our caravan, so that if we did encounter bad weather where we happened to be staying, we could give ourselves and the dogs a bit more shelter. Both suppliers knew our circumstances and worked extremely hard to make sure everything was done prior to us leaving. We had friends and family who were going to water our gardens, collect our mail and generally keep an eye on our house, given it was going to be empty for three months.

Treatment day came around, and as was now the routine, we saw Tim first to go through the scan in detail. The cancer was still asleep, but the main tumour on his heart had not shrunk any further. This meant that the monthly treatment was still holding it at bay but not getting rid of it completely. I remember feeling a little disappointed that it hadn't shrunk. In my mind I was hoping it would just disappear completely. I knew this to be unrealistic, but I am a big believer in miracles. Tim went through where Rod was having treatment while we were traveling and was happy that everything seemed organized. He wished us well. It felt odd, the thought of not seeing him or his team for three months. They had become our security blanket and part of our lives.

With Rod's November treatment done, and the caravan packed, we returned home to spend a few days catching up with friends. On the Saturday morning, with the dogs on the backseat and our caravan behind us, we set off for our holiday odyssey.

CHAPTER FIVE: THE MEMORIES WE MADE

Travelling across Australia meant that we had to drive over 4000 km each way. We wanted to break that up so Rod could rest and recuperate along the way. We had some time up our sleeves before we caught up with Kate, Kev and the girls. We left on the 11th of November and were due to arrive in Eden NSW on the 16th of December. During this time Rod would need to stop and have his first treatment at Port Pirie Hospital in South Australia. We decided that we would push along a bit to get to the other side of the Nullabor and head to a place called Streaky Bay where we would stay for two weeks. From there we would make our way to Port Pirie for treatment on the fifth.

The first three days we only stopped to sleep. It felt nice to be on the road again, we had done this trip many times before, while we were working in the eastern states of Australia. This time would be different, we weren't on a tight deadline. I was worried that the driving would tire Rod too much, but he kept assuring me he was okay. On the second night we stayed behind a roadhouse on the Nullabor, sheltering from the wind. I would look up at the stars, so bright out in the middle of nowhere with no other lights around. I find stars in the night sky fascinating and beautiful, and feel a strong pull towards the Universe that I believe connects us all. I often find myself wondering about other galaxies, life forms even, and whether they are out there looking back at us.

It felt so good to be away from the towns and cities, surrounded only by trees in the middle of nowhere. I had a sense of freedom that I hadn't experienced in a long time. Everything out there seemed so much more vivid. The colours were brighter, the view so much clearer. Where we stayed the next night, however, was a completely different story - a barren landscape of limestone and dust. The wind was so strong, as it blew across from the Great Australian Bight only a few kilometers away, that I struggled to open the caravan door. Rod, the two dogs and I sheltered as best as we could as a lightening storm rolled across the plain and the wind howled; we didn't get much sleep. I was worried this was too much for Rod, but the next morning we pushed on.

We reached Ceduna in South Australia the next day, successfully crossing the Nullabor, wind-blown and exhausted but okay. We had three days booked in a caravan park in Ceduna to allow Rod time to rest and recuperate before we headed to Streaky Bay, a couple of hours south. It's usually the week after each chemo treatment that Rod finds his energies levels slipping. This can last anything from two or three days to a week before he starts to pick up again. I could see he was tired, and with the wind not giving up anytime soon our nights were restless and sleep broken. We kept telling ourselves the wind would drop soon. Unfortunately, it never did.

We arrived in Streaky Bay, where we would take the boat off the roof and do some fishing. All along the way, feathers were appearing right in front of me, and I felt comforted and reassured that spirit was with us, protecting us on our journey. On reflection, I look back now and laugh. I think they were urging me to be patient, as the wind continued for weeks on end. One thing we hadn't realised was that November on the Eyre Peninsula in SA was humorously called "Blow-Vember" and I now understand why. The winds certainly didn't make ideal conditions for fishing, with Rod only getting out on the water one day. I was disappointed for him. This was supposed to be his reward for all the hard work he had done with the treatment this past year. Obviously, the Universe had other plans.

After twelve days of gale force winds and with me becoming ill with what we believe to be a kidney stone, we packed up, put the boat back on the roof, and moved onto Port Pirie in readiness for his next treatment. Port Pirie was a pleasant surprise for us. We had never been there before, and during the few days leading up to treatment we managed to brace the wind and got out and about sightseeing. We scoped out the hospital and where Rod would have blood tests, and felt comfortable knowing where to go. This is one thing we have found through this journey; to reduce the overwhelm of not knowing what to expect, it was important for Rod to see where he needed to be before the appointment day.

The day of treatment we arrived at the hospital, and, as usual, he had an oncology appointment first, before heading to the ward. It all went very smoothly. Being a regional hospital and just five minutes from the caravan park, meant I could leave Rod there, do our shopping and fuel up the car in preparation for the next leg of our trip. We were both relieved when that day was over and happy with how easy it seemed.

As we headed further east, getting closer each day to Kate, Kev and the girls, we managed to spend a couple of days with our friends, Janette and Paul, whom we hadn't seen for a while. A year or so prior, Paul also had cancer treatment for sarcoma. Whilst his was different to Rod's, both he and Janette understand how difficult this journey can be and how important it is to live completely in this moment. When I look back on these couple of days, I feel a sense of warmth that no matter how long between our catch ups, it feels like no time has passed and we feel lucky to have them in our lives. Wishing we could stay longer but with me longing desperately to get to Kate, we said our goodbyes.

Kate knew we were going to be a week ahead of schedule, so we agreed to meet early in Bega NSW, where we would surprise the granddaughters. I don't know who was more anxious that day, me or Kate. I had been holding on so tightly all year, pushing down how much I wanted to see her in the flesh, hold her in a big hug, and every kilometer closer we got, the more emotional I became. We had planned that we would park outside where we were staying and walk in. Kate would get the girls to come outside, saying she had a surprise for them, while she took a video of our reunion. Kate was documenting their own holiday odyssey through her Instagram, the_sandy_tales.

This still brings me to tears when I recall their squeals of delight and Hannah, the youngest, launching herself into my arms, while Layla went straight to her grandpa and trying to hold back her own tears. Hugging Kate and Kev felt like I was home. We were with them all now, and I could finally relax for the first time in nearly twelve months. Being with them felt so right. Layla became my shadow those first few days. Our caravans parked side by side, she would open her bunk window in the morning, see me sitting outside having coffee, and in a quiet voice say, "Morning Nanna," before quickly getting dressed to come sit with us. My heart was overflowing with love, our travels with them just beginning.

Kate's birthday was a beautiful day. Kev had chosen all her presents and bought some decorations which we put up under our awning late the night before, ready to surprise her. We had to keep Kate distracted while we decorated the awning, blew up balloons and prepared for her birthday breakfast. When she came over to our van the next morning, the look on her face told us this was exactly how she wanted to spend her day. We had an amazing lunch at a restaurant in the next town, and spent the rest of the day relaxing by the ocean. I was so grateful that we were with her on this special day, being her 40th birthday, something when Rod was first diagnosed, we weren't sure would happen. Rod even managed to get the boat in the water and he, Kev and Kate spent a fabulous day fishing, with Kate holding the record for most fish that day. Rod and I had picked up six dozen unshucked frozen oysters on our way over from South Australia, to share with them. South Australia is renowned for being the oyster capital of Australia and, in my opinion, they're the largest with the creamiest taste. But as Kate said, after a few weeks of eating oysters she was becoming half human, half oyster, so the fish they caught was a welcome relief.

The days rolled on and we moved to another state, Victoria, where we spent Christmas in a place called Marlo. This is where the Snowy River meets the ocean. The weather was still not being overly kind. Christmas in Australia is supposed to be hot and the best time of the year. It is summer in our hemisphere and when most of us spend time at the beach or outdoors. This Christmas, however, we were in for torrential rain and wind, and with the wild weather forecast we were nervous about how our Christmas lunch would go. Nonetheless, we decorated the annex, set a Christmas table on our camp tables, complete with decorations I had brought from home, and cooked the ham, a turkey roll and made salads. It was a far different Christmas from the one Rod and I had spent last year, alone, in shock and trying to process the fact that he had a tumour. Here we were, one year on and celebrating how far he had come. The weather gods shined down on us that day, and while it did rain and the annex flooded after lunch which made us retreat to our individual caravans, the worst of the weather went around us. The next day it cleared up and the sun appeared once more.

We left Marlo and stayed at a free camp, I say that with tongue in cheek, at a winery near Lakes Entrance. Although it is free, they do like you to either buy a bottle of wine or have lunch at their restaurant. Needless to say, by the time we left there were many bottles of wine in our caravan to bring home, and I think Rod had put on a couple of kilograms after all the lunches there. It was such a peaceful place to stay, and we lit a fire at night to sit out under the stars, drink a few glasses of red wine amongst the trees with a vineyard as our view.

We pushed on to Melbourne for Rod's next treatment, and Kev went into the city with Rod. I was nervous being back in a big city, Covid had reared its ugly head again, with Melbourne being a hotspot. To keep Rod as safe from infection as we could, we were back to wearing masks when we went to shopping centres. We both had big cars which were hard to park in cities, so we were looking for the best option of transport. We decided that it would be too risky to use public transport, so we booked an Uber for them. Both Kev and Rod were disappointed when St. Vincent's Hospital would only let Rod into the treatment room due to the high Covid numbers. But Kev's disappointment was over quickly when he realised he could happily have a pint in a local pub while he waited, much to Rod's disgust.

The caravan park was close to the city, but far enough out to be surrounded with the most amazing scenery and lots of walking trails. One morning I suggested that it might be nice to have a walk with the dogs, and Kev, Kate and the girls agreed. I had walked part of the trail the day before and didn't think it was that long. Leaving Rod at the caravan park, we set off, only for it to turn into a seven km walk, which Kev said felt like a trek, given the track became very narrow and overgrown with trees and bushes.

It seemed like our time in Melbourne flew past, and we were unsure which way we would head next. With it being school holidays in Australia, and the coastal region caravan parks already heavily booked, we decided to head inland and "chase the Murray River out of Victoria" as Kev says. The Murray River is one of the largest in Australia and winds its way through three states with many camping spots along the way. We were hoping it would be slightly quieter than along the coast. We headed to a town called Euchuca, the home of many paddle steamers, which used to be the main way of trading in the 1800s and early 1900s. I was excited by this; I had always wanted to do a trip on the Murray River on a paddle steamer. There were a few to choose from, but we settled on one that would take a one-hour trip upriver during the day. The girls were as excited as I was. At the time when I first booked it, I thought Kate wasn't all that keen about the paddle steamer, but when we arrived and boarded it, the smile on her face told me just how much she was loving it. It was like stepping back in time and getting a glimpse into what Australia must have been like then. Much slower and steadier, taking time to get between towns, the paddle steamers stopped at various properties, dropped off supplies, enjoyed cups of tea and scones before slowly making their way further up or down stream. I reflected that this life would have been far different from the fast paced, technological world we live in today.

It was also in Euchuca where I had a massive meltdown. We were going to a restaurant for dinner and Rod was struggling with walking distances, so it was suggested that we ride Kev and Kate's bikes with the girls, and they would walk across the bridge and into town. I wasn't keen on this idea, I said I was happy to walk, and the others could ride. In the end I lost the battle and proceeded to get on the bike. Now, when Rod rides a bike, I'm sure he thinks he is competing in the Tour de France and, off he went with Layla in tow. Hannah and I were struggling to keep up, it was a very hot day, and I was sweating profusely when I caught up to him. My shorts were soaking. I thought this was sweat, but I later discovered that Kate's seat had gotten very wet with all the rain, and it was the water seeping out of the sponge. I had a huge breakdown, about how I didn't want to ride in the first place; I would have to go back and get changed; that Kate's bike was awful; that Rod had just ridden off and left us so we had to peddle harder to catch up. It wasn't pretty and even though I knew my inner child was playing up, I couldn't calm her down.

Layla, in the meantime, was trying to hold back her laughter, while Hannah was trying to support me, saying, "Yes, Grandpa, we couldn't keep up, I'm exhausted and now look at Nanna's shorts," Layla assured me that if I pulled my shirt out it would cover my shorts, and no one would think I had wet myself. I proceeded to walk the rest of the way to the restaurant, with Rod trying to dodge the sharp glares I was sending him. When Kate and Kev caught up to us, Layla couldn't wait to tell them that "Nanna had a tantrum" and she had never seen me do that before. She was laughing so much that it set Kate off laughing, and in the end we were all laughing so hard we were crying. Layla now teases me when she can see I'm getting stressed, asking if I'm about to have another tantrum, which quickly stops me in my tracks. Euchuca turned out to be one of the highlights of our trip and we all enjoyed our time there.

We weren't sure where we were headed next as we were getting close to leaving Kate, Kev and the girls, and I found myself consumed with researching which towns Rod and I would explore and which caravan parks to stay in. Constantly changing my mind about our plans, I had so wanted to just go with the flow on this journey, but that wasn't easy for me. I knew this was starting to frustrate not only Rod, but Kate and Kev as well. I was angry at myself, why couldn't I just decide and stick with it? I felt like I was spending so much time planning that I was forgetting the whole purpose of our trip was to make memories and to have fun. I talked this over with Kate, who is my voice of reason, and also a social worker, so she's no stranger to dealing with people experiencing trauma and emotional overwhelm. You would think as a counsellor I would have been all over this myself, but it was after a conversation with Kate I had the ah-ha moment. I realised that for some people who have experienced trauma, it's necessary to have structure and concrete plans, and that going with the flow felt unsafe. As a counsellor, I would often explain this to my clients, that if structure feels safer for them, that's perfectly okay. Now, I'm not saying we don't live in the moment, because we do, but to have a plan which takes the stress off and gives us something to move towards was highly beneficial for me. With this new awareness of myself, and with Kate's help, I booked our next few caravan parks and got back to enjoying our time together.

Our days in Euchuca came to an end, and it was time to leave Kate, Kev and the girls and start making our way west. We wanted to visit the Barossa Valley, one of our wine regions in South Australia on our way back, whereas they wanted to keep chasing the Murray River, so we tearfully said goodbye. Layla was begging us to stay with them, but I explained that Grandpa needed another treatment, which meant that we had to get back to South Australia. It was extremely hard driving away from them, but grateful for the memories we had made, we moved on.

We spent a wonderful few days in the Barossa Valley in South Australia, which reminded me of my childhood and the time I had spent in the South of France. We had a few beautiful lunches and spent the days touring the countryside surrounded by grape vines. Leaving there, we headed to a town called Port Broughton where we would spend just over a week before Rod's next treatment in Port Pirie. Travelling with dogs in a caravan is not an easy thing to do, especially when one of them is very large and very hairy. Bodhi, our big and older dog, had become quite fearful of not only the wind, but also had become quite reactive to other dogs. This made it hard for us in caravan parks with lots of other dogs around. It was also tiring for both of us as we were constantly on alert to his reactions. We made the decision that when we travel in the future, Bodhi would probably stay home and we would take

Ben, our young Cavoodle, to get him used to travelling without watching Bodhi's reactions to everything. By the time we got to Port Broughton, Bodhi was becoming increasingly hard work, and I was exhausted. Once again, the weather was not our friend, and we were both feeling a little homesick. I was also missing the girls, even though we had only just left them.

We got news from Kate that she had cut her foot in a lake a few days back. It was very swollen, and she was worried it might be infected, so had gone to a district hospital nearby. They were admitting her on intravenous antibiotics. I was concerned about this as I know how quickly infections from cuts can take hold and turn nasty. Being on edge, Rod realised that our plans might have to change quickly. The next day she told us that they had done a scan and there was a foreign body embedded in it. They had tried for over four hours at the local hospital and couldn't get it out under local anesthetic, so they would be transferring her to Royal Adelaide hospital the next day for general surgery. While I was worried for Kate, I felt for Kev; he had the caravan, the two girls and Ned, their dog, to think about while his wife was now on her way to another hospital over an hour away.

We made the decision to turn around and head back to meet Kev in a caravan park that he had managed to book us both into, in Adelaide. That way we could look after the girls and Ned, while he visited Kate. I was also needing to see her myself, in the flesh, so I could reassure myself she was okay. Another trauma response of mine. What we thought was going to be a quick trip in and out of hospital turned into five days, with Kate finally being released to come home with a padded boot while her stitches and foot healed.

Whilst Adelaide was not on our original itinerary, it gave all of us time to look around. The girls' birthdays were coming up and this was the last major city to do some shopping. With Kate in a boot and not walking very far, she asked if I could take them shopping. I took the girls to a nearby shopping centre on a terrible day, weather wise. Torrential rain all day. I was driving the Chevy truck which was hard to park because of its size, so I had to park some distance from the shop entrance. The girls and I got soaked. I could tell that Layla was looking at me to see if one of Nanna's tantrums was coming. Needless to say, on a shopping trip with Nanna, they got thoroughly spoilt.

We celebrated Hannah's ninth birthday in an Italian restaurant just around the corner, and I fell in love with this city. I mentioned to Rod whether he would consider moving here, which was wishful thinking on my behalf or maybe running away from our reality. I could tell his response wasn't the same as mine, so I let that idea drop.

Once again, it was time to say goodbye to them. As we were leaving, Layla said to me, "I told you that you shouldn't have gone, Nanna, and if we were to hurt ourselves would you come back?" I assured her I would come back if any of them hurt themselves, to which she turned to her little sister Hannah and said, "Quick Han, break your leg, so Nanna has to stay." This made us all laugh, especially as it wasn't her getting hurt. I explained to her, through our laughter, that we couldn't come back; Grandpa was close to having treatment and after that we needed to get back to Western Australia. The tears weren't as bad this time, as I knew we would be seeing them again in two months as they made their way back home.

The treatment at Port Pirie didn't go quite to plan. Rod's veins were being difficult, and the nurses had trouble getting a canula in. In the end, they called the surgical anesthetist who finally managed to get a vein. With the final treatment done before the next scan, we moved onto our last stop at Ceduna where we rested for a few days again, before heading back across the Nullabor. I had been having these niggling feelings for the past couple of weeks that we needed to get to the other side of the Nullabor. Those feelings was getting stronger daily. I couldn't explain it other than a deep knowing, and a sense of something going wrong if we didn't. We discussed it, and with Rod getting very tired, having been travelling for three months and my uneasy feeling, we decided that we would cut our trip short and head for home. We didn't know it at the time but thankfully I listened to my intuition, as the week we had originally planned to cross the Nullabor, a large fire was burning out of control, and they closed the road for days on end. This would have meant that Rod would have missed his PET scan and February treatment. Thank you, Universe, for intervening on that one.

We arrived home in Western Australia, with a full heart and lots of wonderful memories.

CHAPTER SIX: THE PAST TWELVE MONTHS

I had been thinking long and hard about where to end this first part of the book and after much consideration, I decided that it would be appropriate to end it as we approached the twelve-month mark since Rod commenced treatment. There is so much that we have both learnt from these past twelve months that I would like to summarise below.

- We have learned many lessons when it comes to travelling with a cancer diagnosis. While we enjoyed our three-month holiday odyssey, on reflection, we would choose shorter time frames to be away from home. For both of us, this extended period away in a caravan became exhausting, where we longed for our own king size bed and the space in the house to move around, especially for the dogs who were tired of being confined in small spaces. Planning was crucial, as was being prepared for plans to change at a moment's notice. I researched where the medical facilities were, and how quickly we could get there if we needed to. We had an email from Tim which outlined Rod's cancer type and the treatment. Giving Tim plenty of time to organize the treatment made the whole process so much easier.

- For me, writing checklists well in advance of what I needed to take with us in case we got stuck anywhere remote, made it easier when it came time to pack. We learnt quickly that next time we would consider not travelling during peak periods, especially school holidays, because with the increased numbers in the caravan parks came the risk of infection. For Rod, we would try to do things in the morning, so that he could have a rest each afternoon and be mindful how far he had to walk due to neuropathy in his feet.

- It has been important for me to honour my own journey as much as Rod's, throughout this process. As much as I would like life to return to normal, as with any traumatic event, there can be no going back to our old life. I now recognize there are always going to be the crappy days, those days when it feels like dark clouds hang over our heads, but I also know that in time those clouds will part and the sun will rise again.

- Moving through the fear and processing this new reality, especially in those first few weeks and months, takes patience and much self-care, even when it feels selfish to do so. Remembering, through all the sadness, that I still had a right to be happy, smile and laugh.
- Understanding all the medical terminology was crucial for me, especially when it came to reading scan results and treatment options. Asking Tim for clarification of things if I was unsure what something meant, helped demystify the jargon.
- Learning to let Rod just be! That was the hardest lesson, trying not to control everything for him. Remembering and respecting him as an individual and being perfectly capable of making his own decisions, even when I wasn't happy with them.
- Living completely in the moment, whether that be a good day or bad day, and not suppressing my own emotions because they make others feel uncomfortable or unsure how to respond.
- Dealing with the scanxiety in the week leading up to the PET scan, by journaling, distraction, plenty of meditation and breathwork to help settle my nervous system.

So, in conclusion of this chapter, Rod's PET scan was scheduled for the 26th of February. Instead of our normal accommodation, which is at one of the two Cancer Council lodges here in Western Australia, I thought it would be nice if we could stay closer to the ocean and in a hotel, where we could go for lunch and dinner after his scan. The past twelve months had been consumed with his diagnosis and treatment, and this year we were more determined than ever to live our lives alongside his diagnosis, and honour our relationship as a couple. I booked our hotel room, overlooking the ocean where I thought we could watch the sunset on the beach and sit in those moments of silent reflection, grateful for everything we do have in our life, rather than focus on everything we don't have.

However, once again, the Universe had other plans. I like to draw an oracle card each morning, asking what my soul needs to know today. I had been drawing uncomfortable cards, indicating that there was change coming and a hurdle to overcome. Now, my first thought was this was to do with Rod and his upcoming scan, but three days out from Rod's scan our old dog, Bodhi, became quite ill. He had a bacterial infection in his ear, the worst one the vet had ever seen. He also has spinal degeneration and getting his pain under control has been difficult. He was very ill, and I knew that we couldn't leave him with our friend, Mandy, who would pet, and house sit for us, so I cancelled our hotel booking and we decided to drive up and back for the scan on the Monday, and then back up again on the Wednesday for results and treatment.

Additionally, the few days leading up to Rod's scan I was more anxious than usual, interestingly not because of Rod's scan but because my brother, Steve, was undergoing his own cancer surgery - a diagnosis that had shocked us in the days before Christmas 2023. Rod's cancer diagnosis was Christmas 2022, and my father had died on Christmas Day in 2011. Christmas is supposed to be a time of joy, but I was starting to question my beliefs around this now. I was worried about my brother, feeling a little triggered by everything that was going on for him. A few weeks prior, I lost my beloved Aunt Pauline, who lived in the UK. We had spent a great deal of time with each other when I was in my early twenties when she lived in Australia, and I thought of her more of a sister than an aunt.

As is our normal routine, Rod started his no carb diet the day before the scan, and underwent the sixteen hours of fasting. Monday morning, we drove to Perth, where he had his PET scan and we returned home to look after Bodhi. We distracted ourselves the best we could on Tuesday, and later that evening we watched my aunt's funeral via live stream. It was an emotional night, but I was extremely grateful for technology and being able to say our goodbyes, albeit through a computer screen.

Wednesday morning, I felt very calm. I had been reflecting on this for a few days, that I wasn't concerned about these results. It was as if my soul knew that it was going to be okay. But there was still that moment of anxious waiting in Tim's rooms, and we let out a huge sigh of relief when Tim welcomed us back with the news that the cancer was still stable. Tim said that if we wanted to continue travelling, this would be possible. We spoke about where we could go, and that if we wanted to travel overseas it would be better if we visited countries with reciprocal medical agreements. Tim told us that with Rod's type of cancer there is no way of knowing whether Rod will live six months, twelve months or two years, and that while he is still well enough to do so, we should live our lives as best we can. We talked much about how we call it living our lives alongside cancer, not dying it from it.

I often talk about how we live our lives in three-month blocks, from scan to scan, and I talk about this further in part two of the book, but for now Rod and I continue to remain committed to each other as a couple, to live our lives now, to love and enjoy our time together no matter how long that may be. We'll continue to integrate his cancer diagnosis into our lives and continue to make as many memories as we can.

We have lots to look forward to, as we celebrate our fifteenth wedding anniversary in April and have lots of small trips planned.

At the time of completing this part of the book Rod's cancer is still asleep.

Part II

MY PERSONAL JOURNEY

"I honour my soul and my own journey through this chapter in our lives."

I've spent the better part of the fifteen months since Rod's diagnosis reflecting on this journey, and through this part of the book, I hope to share with you a collection of my emotions and experiences. I promised myself I would be authentic and vulnerable and show you, the reader, that any emotions and feelings you may be experiencing are a normal part of the process, and encourage you to be gentle with yourself. I have written these in no chronological order, but to simply to share with you my recollections and journal entries over this time.

I would also like to share with you what I've learnt about myself; how much I've grown spiritually and emotionally; how to move forward when it feels like your world is crumbling around you and give you a glimmer of hope that you, too, are much stronger than you realise.

I am a huge advocate for self-reflection as a way of healing and I do this regularly through my journaling and my writing. The reflections within these chapters are designed to support you, as well providing me with an outlet for processing my own trauma.

I want you to know that you are not alone, and hope you find some comfort in reading about my personal journey.

> "Our stories may be similar, our journeys different, but in this moment, I see you and recognise you in me."

THE FIRST FEW DAYS & WEEKS

I remember those first few days and weeks as if I was watching a movie play out before me. The shock of hearing the news about the suspicious mass, not knowing what it was, but my own intuition telling me it was something very serious, was almost too much to bear. I alternated between crying and trying to be supportive, whilst trying to live life as normal. My mind was in overdrive, and I felt like I was constantly asking Rod if he was okay. Wanting to know what he was thinking, trying to gauge what was going on for him.

No one can prepare you for how you are going to react in this moment. There were times I felt almost hysterical, laughing at nothing, and then dissolving into tears. Other times were like I was in slow motion, as if someone had slowed down the movie so that you can see every tiny detail. There were days when I felt numb, like I was having an out of body experience.

I wasn't functioning well at all. I couldn't even start to contemplate what we were having for dinner, let alone do any housework. The dogs weren't getting walked and my own self-care went out the window. I was consumed with guilt. Guilt that I might say the wrong thing. Guilt that Rod would read my thoughts. Guilt that it wasn't me going through this. I know that sounds strange, but I liken it to survivor's guilt. Two people in a relationship, one suddenly gets ill and unsure how long their life will be or dies suddenly, whilst the other's life goes on, feeling guilty that they get to live. I have dealt with this many times with clients in my former counselling practice and now, here I was, experiencing similar emotions myself.

My normally positive, upbeat self was nowhere to be found. Instead, it was replaced with an angry, frustrated, sad shell of a person I didn't recognize. I was angry with the medical system, frustrated that things weren't moving quickly enough, and worried that as each day passed, the tumour could be growing and spreading. We spent a great deal of time waiting for medical professionals to contact us and each day felt like an eternity.

The biggest thing for me was the fear - fear that comes with being told this. I kept thinking I was going to lose Rod. I tried my hardest to stay positive, but I just couldn't. There were so many tearful phone conversations with my family and friends, who tried desperately to cheer me up. Nothing helped. It was a grief like I had never experienced before. The sense of disbelief, this isn't happening to us. It happens to others, but not us. My husband can't possibly have cancer. They have it wrong, how could they get it so wrong? Yet deep down I knew what they were telling us was very real, which made the sense of helplessness and spinning out of control worse.

The smallest of things creep in, thoughts that don't even mean anything in the big scheme of life. I was thinking, we haven't even done the renovations to the kitchen yet. The carport has to be rebuilt; how would we get that done with him being sick? How would I cope with this house if Rod died? What about the holidays we had booked? All meaningless on reflection, but at that point your mind isn't in the right place to think rationally or logically.

I completely lost my empathy for other people. When anyone would start talking about their struggles or issues, all I could think was, *is it really that big of a deal? At least you're not going through what I'm going through - my husband has cancer!* I would become frustrated with people taking up too much of my time, when all I wanted to do was wallow in my own sadness. My trauma seemed so much worse than anyone else's in those moments. As a counsellor, I often explain to people that each person's definition of trauma is relevant to their own lived experience. What might seem traumatic for one person may just be a blip on the radar for another. Everyone's experience is valid and not to be discounted, so when I started discounting other people's experiences, I felt awful, and it was as if all my years of training went out the window. I was grateful that I had my journal to write my thoughts into and to process my own emotions and guilt.

There was so much to do in those early days, with running to and from appointments, sometimes leaving home before dawn, so totally exhausted when you finally return that you just want to flop into a chair and not move. The thought of cooking dinner almost too much, yet knowing that we needed to keep the nutrition up to help us sustain this long term. At times, I couldn't even remember what day it was let alone what needed to be done. I pushed the bills to one side, telling myself I would pay them later, only to realise that I hadn't. I became clingy with

Rod, wanting to be as close to him as possible, yet the sadness I was exuding must have been painful for him to cope with.

My sister, Ann, and brother-in-law, Chris, met us at the hospital for the first few appointments when Rod was due for a scan, something I was extremely grateful for. When you're waiting on your own, sitting in a coffee shop, tears streaming down your face, it can feel so lonely, while at the same time not wanting to make eye contact with anyone in case they asked you if you were okay. So having them with me helped keep me distracted, and I felt that I could cry if I wanted to because they were there to shelter me. But as time went on, the scan days, even through the scanxiety, got easier and I began to occupy myself with reading or writing.

In those early days, the initial shock and trauma were something that I needed to work through and there was no shortcutting the process. It's painful and messy, there's no magic way to move through this, nor a protocol to follow. All I can tell you is that as the weeks drew on, and we started the process of full diagnosis and treatment, the shock started to settle, and life began to take on its own form. Routines started appearing and things that once seemed foreign and scary became familiar, and in some ways comforting. The worry and fear were still there, but coping mechanisms appeared along way. Seeking support quickly in those early days would have made my process easier, yet I waited until we were well into the diagnosis stage.

I knew this was going to be a very long journey, and somehow I had to find a way to navigate my own way through it, just as Rod was navigating his own way through his personal experience.

I began journaling more than usual. Every time I felt like I couldn't do this, I would get out my journal and write. I would write about how sad I felt, how unfair life was. I would write about my anger and how I just wanted to scream and run away, tell everyone to leave me alone and not give me advice, even if it was well-meaning. Then eventually, when I had written all the negative emotions - getting them out of my head, which felt so much better - I would ask myself what my soul needed from me that day. As I kept writing, I found that I became softer and kinder to myself and others. I would lean into the feelings, instead of pushing them away. The more I wrote, the more I could understand myself.

I also used distraction a lot in those early days. Not to hide from my reality, but to keep my overthinking mind to my journal where I could safely process my emotions. I started to de-clutter the house which also helped with clearing the negative energy. At first though, I packed up my beautiful sound bowls and put them away, thinking I will never use them again. I felt that holistic part of my life was over. But my good friend, Jodi, begged me not to sell them. A counsellor herself, she recognized what I was going through and knew that what I needed in that moment was not to make drastic changes in my life in one swoop. I wasn't thinking clearly, and putting them away helped me to not think too far into the future, and just focus on what was happening today.

I love breathwork, I use it every day. It is one of the most powerful tools to help with reducing stress and anxiety. It doesn't matter what breathwork technique you try, just mastering the way to breathe deeply and slowly into your chest and abdomen, and then releasing the breath even more slowly, automatically calms your nervous system. When you do this in repetition, you find you can stop anxiety and panic attacks in their tracks. Your whole body softens, and it allows more oxygen to flow through your blood stream. Breathwork while standing up, especially barefooted, helps to keep you grounded in this moment.

KEEP YOUR CHIN UP

I want to let you know that I am a big believer in the power of positive thinking and am always looking for ways to provide support, but one of the things I found difficult at the start of this journey was when people told me to "keep my chin up". I got to the stage where I wanted to scream at them. As a counsellor, those words make me cringe at the best of times, but as the partner of someone who has just been diagnosed with cancer, keeping my chin up was the last thing I felt like I could do.

People mean well when they say these things, it's something we've heard many times as words of encouragement, but it's just not that helpful, in my opinion, to the person going through difficult times. But being the person I am, instead of screaming, I just smiled and said thanks.

There are many other things people say, "It's going to be okay; he can beat this, you need to stay positive, and the treatment will work, trust me." These are all words I have had said to me. What I found though, is that instead of bringing comfort I went further into myself, retreating from people, at the same time thinking, "It's not okay, how do you know it's going to work?" I used to teach people how to support and communicate effectively with others in times of difficulty and look at some of the more helpful things to say, so I knew I was being a bit cold when these unhelpful words were being said to me. I would release my frustration in my journal, often writing about how invalidated I felt. It was like my fears and emotions were not allowed and I needed to shut them down.

"Stay positive," they would say. In those early days of shock and trauma, how does one stay positive, when you have no idea if the person you love is going to live or die? I even heard it said to Rod or written on his Facebook posts, "You've got this, Rod." Yet when I looked at him knowing there was a six-centimeter monster attached to his heart and growing daily, I knew he had anything but "got this".

As with all the positive words of encouragement, everyone had their own story to share of someone they knew who had cancer, how they overcame it, or didn't overcome it. Sometimes I would listen, trying to understand why they were telling me this, but all too often, I found it all too overwhelming, not wanting to hear about other people's circumstances. I didn't want to hear about people who didn't survive which was just a reminder that I was facing the reality of losing Rod. I was too consumed in my own grief to find this helpful.

I spent many hours reflecting on this, and what I realised is when you are trying to process this type of trauma, it's important to find your voice and the space to express your emotions and feelings freely, without feeling shut down. I started creating healthy boundaries with others by explaining that as much as they mean well by saying these words, for me they didn't feel comforting or reassuring, and that one of the things I needed most in this moment was for them to simply listen to me, to hold space for me rather than try to tell me it was going to be okay, because at that point no one knew it was going to be okay. The last thing I wanted was for people to try to give me hope when there may not have been any.

Through my own self-reflection I knew that I had to go a layer deeper. I had to explore what was underneath my anger and frustration at hearing these words. I know that anger wasn't the primary emotion and through my reflection it was the feeling that my fears and concerns weren't valid or important. It felt like I was being asked to mask what I was truly feeling, which in turn made me feel guilty for not being positive, and feeling judged that they might be thinking I was giving up on Rod.

The same went for how I was communicating with Rod. It can be hard to support your partner when you're falling apart yourself. Just as people meant well with me, I also fell into the trap of doing the same with Rod, yet initially I couldn't bring myself to say anything that would give him false hope until we knew much more about what we were dealing with.

Rod can find it hard to communicate his feelings, so when I fell into the trap of asking him closed questions such as "are you feeling okay?", I got a yes or no answer. This would just leave me frustrated that he wasn't letting me in. I knew I had to tackle this another way, so I put on my counsellor hat and began to ask him open questions and phrases such as:

"That news must have been hard to hear. What are your thoughts on it?"

"The treatment sounds like it's going to be tough. What concerns do you have?"

"What can we do that will make the waiting easier until the test results are completed?"

"What is something we can do to ease the stress you might be feeling right now?"

"How are you truly feeling behind the 'I'm doing OK?'"

"I'm scared about this but I'm right here with you every step of the way, you're not alone."

When I did this, I found he became more open with me and the communication between us improved, which in turn deepened the connection we had with each other. It felt like we were in this together and somehow together we could get through this, whilst at the same time being open and authentic with our feelings. Now that we are well into this journey, I find it easier when people use words of encouragement. I still smile and thank them, knowing that they mean well. But what I have learnt about people in general, is that most don't know how to hold space for another or have the right words to say. So, they say, "it's going to be okay."

TELLING FAMILY AND FRIENDS

In the beginning, when we first heard that Rod needed an internal heart ultrasound, although I felt uneasy I wasn't locked in fear. I thought that the worst-case scenario might be that Rod would need heart surgery. It was easy to communicate this to family and friends.

But when the shock came and we learnt there was a tumour, we were plunged into who to tell, how much to tell and when to tell. I instantly told our immediate family and closest friends, but we held off telling the granddaughters. We didn't feel they needed the worry at this stage. Making the phone calls and endless texts was extremely difficult. We both felt that we were telling the same story over and over. Each time it got bigger and scarier in our minds. I started to forget what I had already told people.

My brain was foggy, and I found I was repeating myself over and over with the same person. This is a common trauma response and happens to many people. When you experience trauma, symptoms some people may experience include brain fog, which I describe as a heaviness in my head, not remembering where things are or what I have already told someone; while others may experience being unable to speak clearly, or completely shut down not speaking at all; while still others find their words are coming out extremely fast and almost non-coherent. Trauma affects everyone differently, there is no one size fits all approach when trying to understand what trauma looks like.

When all the tests were starting, it seemed like the more messages we were receiving. It was only natural that people wanted to know how Rod was doing and what was going on, but it felt like our phones were going nonstop, and each time we repeated the story we were becoming more traumatised ourselves. It felt like there was no escaping this nightmare. We talked through about how we could keep everyone informed and in the loop, except for close family and friends whom we communicated with regularly. As I have a business social media page, we decided that we would turn that into a cancer blog which would allow us to share our journey as well as keep everyone updated with Rod's scans, treatment, and other information.

We talked through what we would post and how much we wanted

people to know. This worked well for us. I have had many of Rod's friends reach out and tell me how they look for my posts, it keeps them all informed with the same information at the same time. When it comes to the grandchildren, we were still hesitant to use the word cancer. We talked about his treatment and that he's still sick. At first, we told them there was a risk he might not get better, but we left out all the other details unless they specifically asked.

The hardest thing I found was running into people in our local shops, who would ask me how I was doing. I could relay all the information on what was going on with Rod, but when it came to how I was doing, I would crumble and dissolve into tears. I recognised I had been on autopilot, that I was disassociating from my own emotions until faced with being asked the questions about myself. Instead of processing my own trauma, I started avoiding people. I began online shopping so that I didn't run into anyone I knew. I would write my posts on social media which enabled me to still communicate with people, but at a distance. It was easier for me because I could hide behind the screen and not reveal truly how I was doing. Was this healthy? Probably not, but in those early days it was necessary for me, and I'm a big advocate for knowing what is best for you in that moment.

Eventually, I acknowledged that hiding from the world wasn't healthy in the long run. I started to work on processing my own trauma. I was writing in my journal daily, writing how I was feeling each day. I have found that we often get pushed into doing things that other people feel is best for us, going along with it because we are so confused ourselves and doubting or double guessing what we need, but in reality I found it important to give myself the space to ask the question each day, "What will make me feel more comfortable right now?" I spent time doing breathwork and taking time throughout my day to check in with my body, as to how I was feeling in that moment.

I allowed myself to cry, and set boundaries around how long I would stay in those sad moments. Acknowledging my fears helped me to face them. I recognized that each day would be different. Different fears and emotions would come up, but instead of bundling them into one big pile of trauma, I picked just one to address at a time. I would validate my fear, acknowledging its presence. I would often ask myself it if it was something I needed to focus on in this moment or was this something that could wait until later when we had more information, or I had the time to process it further. Additionally, I would challenge myself whether this fear was real or unfounded and I would ask it, what it was trying to tell me.

Often, our fears are just the body's and mind's way of trying to keep us safe. But when fear arises, it can be so overwhelming that it can feel impossible to find a way forward. So, I would ask myself, what *else in that moment could I do to help me to feel safe*, looking for alternatives and options. Doing all of this helped me to face people again and I began to feel stronger when someone rang, or I would run into someone in the street who we knew.

PLANNING FOR THE FUTURE

When we first knew there was a tumour and even before the actual diagnosis, we recognised that there might be a risk of Rod dying or becoming very ill. One of the things we didn't have in place was an up-to-date Will, and all our vehicles and caravans were in Rod's name only. This made me feel very nervous. I wasn't thinking clearly, my father had died very quickly after his diagnosis of mesothelioma, and I was worried this might happen to Rod. Now, some of you might think I was writing him off and pre-empting something that might not happen, but when you're faced with this situation your brain isn't thinking logically.

I was frightened to tell Rod that I wanted to update our Wills and transfer the vehicles into my name, but I worried that he might die and I would be left to sort it all out at a time when I should be grieving his loss. I have heard this many times from my clients over the years, that it took them longer to grieve their loss due to the first several months being spent sorting through the paperwork, and that they felt cheated of that time. Not wanting that to happen to me, I approached the subject cautiously. I'm being honest here when I tell you I softened the conversation with Rod, telling him it was important in case something happens to either one of us, which was a real possibility. I didn't want him thinking there was no hope, although deep down I think he knew what my fears were.

We made the appointment with the lawyer quickly, and got it all sorted. We had a new Will prepared for both of us, especially as our circumstances had changed a great deal since the last one; a power of attorney appointed; and an advanced health care plan put in place. It was a huge relief for me to have it done and it felt like both of us had a say in what would happen to us in the future. I then turned my attention to having some of the vehicle registrations transferred into my name. This would make it easier if Rod deteriorated suddenly and I had to sell one of the vehicles.

I spoke to our friend, Kay, about the overwhelm of trying to transfer the vehicles into my name. What would normally seem like a straightforward thing to do, suddenly felt very complicated and frustrating. I didn't have the emotional energy to figure it out. Let me tell you about Kay... she is one of the kindest people I know, who would do anything for you in a heartbeat and her way of showing love is through acts of service. She immediately jumped into gear and offered to get that organised for me. This was not easy, as we had a caravan that we bought in another state of Australia which was still registered there. This needed to be changed over first, before it could then be changed into my name.

Between Kay, her husband, Matt, and another friend, Troy, and with a lot of running around, they managed to have the caravan and the car transferred into my name. I felt such a huge relief and was extremely grateful to them.

Rod's superannuation was another thing we had to look closely at. We found out that in Australia, superannuation companies ask you to reconfirm your beneficiaries every two years. It seemed like suddenly everything we had been putting on the back burner for years had to be done in a hurry, due to the upcoming biopsy surgery. We knew there was risk associated with this procedure because at that time, James, the surgeon had told us if the opportunity arose to remove the tumour, he would do so.

It's my belief that when you receive a diagnosis that could result in death or permanent disability, the last thing you want to spend time doing is putting affairs in order. Instead, taking the time to plan prior, allows you to focus completely on treatment and supporting your loved one - it eases the stress on the family and executors of a Will - and the hardest part is having the conversation. This made me reflect about my own funeral planning, which is something Rod and I had never thought to discuss before. But it had me thinking about planning for myself, once again to take pressure off my family. I am an advocate for pre-planning and if you can, also pre-paying. Nominating who will undertake the ceremony, where you would like it to be, who you would like to speak, if anyone, even down to the type of music you would like played.

I know a lot of people may feel that it doesn't matter after you are gone, but for me, I know that anything I can do to take the pressure off my family through this period, I will do. Having gone through both my parents' funerals, even as a close family there were still moments of tension as we tried to make decisions together. The last thing I would want for my daughter, or Rod, to go through is worrying whether they had planned my funeral as per my wishes. I recognise that this pre-planning isn't always an option when there is a sudden death, and having these conversations with your loved ones can be awkward and uncomfortable, but they're necessary. No one really wants to plan what happens to them after they die, but life is a cycle. We are born and we die. As painful as this is for those left behind, it's a fact of life. No one escapes death and we make lots of plans for our lives and our future, so why then would we not plan for our inevitable death?

I feel the more we remove the stigma of death and dying and embrace the cycle, the easier it will be to allow the grieving process to occur, and for those left behind to move forward with their lives.

OUR FAMILY PHOTO SHOOT

Kate and Kev had bought me a family photo shoot for my 60th birthday, which was in August 2022, four months prior to Rods tumour being discovered. We hadn't decided when we wanted to have this done, thinking there was no hurry. But when we knew what we were dealing with, and with Kate, Kev and the girls planning to head off around Australia for twelve months, we decided to book it in.

Meghan, the photographer, was a friend of Kate's. Some years earlier, Meghan had lost her beautiful little girl, Piper, to a cancer called neuroblastoma. Meghan knew of our situation and having experienced her own trauma and loss, we knew she would be the perfect person to capture our moments. We wanted our photos to reflect our individual personalities and our love of nature, so we arranged for the photos to be taken in a bush setting, in a blend of earthiness and greenery with light and shadow. I reflected on this as being spiritually appropriate, because this was how I felt my life was currently, covered with light and shadow.

We took some time to choose the clothes we would wear. We all wanted to look as natural as possible, not staged and looking nothing like our true selves. In the end, our clothes and colour choices all blended beautifully and we looked just as I had imagined it to be. Individual, but woven together through our earthy colours and textures.

It was a very emotional day for me. I know there were times when both Kate and Kev struggled to hold it together as well. I kept thinking *will this be the last family photo shoot we will ever have?* I cried through some of it, seeing Rod with Kate, Kev and the granddaughters, with them not fully knowing how sick grandpa was, made my heart feel very heavy, yet blessed with the knowledge that we are so lucky to have him in our lives. I thought in that moment, how innocent the girls looked, how happy they were to be having photos taken with us. I did wonder how Rod was feeling about the day, whether he was thinking the same as me. Was he thinking we booked and rushed it through because we feared the worst? If he did, he certainly didn't talk about it with me, instead he just held me while I cried.

Through the sadness, there was also a lot of fun. Kev and Rod were being silly and joking with each other, which made us all laugh. We managed to get some amazing photos and Meghan certainly managed to capture the love that Rod and I have for each other, and the love we have for our family. Afterwards, I felt a sense of comfort knowing we had some fabulous photos of us all. Memories that will stay with us forever, and photos of Rod before chemotherapy began and all that comes with that. I knew that once he started treatment his appearance would change and his hair would disappear, although at that time I had no idea how drastic that change would be.

I look back on these photos often, whilst I see the stress and worry on both our faces, I see a man who had no idea what the future held, a sense of innocence about him. There are days when I wish we could go back to that day. I've heard it from my clients before, that they wish they had more photos of them together and I'm extremely grateful that we have those.

LIFE ON HOLD

One of the hardest struggles I found, especially with Kate, Kev and the girls leaving on their year long trip around Australia, was my jealousy of their freedom and how much my own life was on hold. I was sad that she wasn't going to be here with me, sad that it wasn't us going. Even though we had talked it through and encouraged them to go, I knew it was going to be hard on me. Kate, Kev, and the girls are my life, and not being able to go and stay with them or give them a hug was a painful thought. Whilst video calls are good, they're not the same, and holding on for twelve months until they returned home seemed like an eternity.

2023 was supposed to be a year filled with lots of small trips for Rod and me. We had so many plans, then life, in an instant, was suddenly on hold. I was frustrated and confused with trying to make daily decisions, let alone ones for the future and I found myself putting decisions off. Shall we do the kitchen renovations? What if he gets sicker, we don't want contractors in the house while he's resting. Is it worth spending any more money on the caravan or car if we can't travel? All these thoughts were going through my mind.

I wanted to fly to Queensland to see my friend, Vicki, but I didn't want to leave Rod in case he got an infection whilst I wasn't there, and I was fearful that something would happen to him with me on the other side of Australia. Then came the guilt for wanting to go and see her, feeling selfish that I needed to be with my friend when he was going through so much. I pushed away all thoughts of visiting and made excuses that the timing always seemed to be wrong.

In those very early days, Rod was having trouble making commitments for the future. He takes a long time to process anything new at the best of times, and now he was three times worse. I realised, after talking it through with him, he had been hoping for surgery and therefore didn't want to make any plans. When surgery was ruled out, he began to be more open to planning for the future.

I'm the impulsive one in the relationship, and once I get my mind and heart set on something I go after it with everything I've got. Rod is my stabiliser. I was frustrated, deflated, and felt trapped at home. So, when Kate and Kev left, I started watching for their regular updates on social media. I was so happy for them, but inside I was screaming that should be us! I remember sitting in the hospital garden outside the chemo suite sobbing because they were in the Kimberley in Western Australia, a place I always wanted to go with Rod, yet here I was waiting for my husband to finish his weekly treatment.

I began to hate the house, it was no longer my sanctuary, and now felt like my prison. I would stand at our lounge window looking out at our caravan and cry, wondering if we would ever get to use it again. I became so bad, I wanted to move it and store it somewhere else - out of sight, out of mind. The following is an excerpt from my journal one rainy dismal day.

> I sit and listen to the rain as it beats down on our tin roof. Life feels heavy and ready to burst, like the clouds above. The tears fall silently down my cheeks. They symbolise a release, a cleansing. A cleansing of the earth of my soul, just as the rain cleanses the ground beneath my feet. In this moment I allow myself to feel the pain, the sorrow, the regret. I think of a life that could be, one that is not on hold. One that is waiting for us on the other side of this hell. What will become of us I wonder, where is this journey leading us. There is no answer for my questions today, so I sit and listen to the soft rainfall instead. The rain outside and the rainfall deep within my soul.

We had sold our Mandurah house in June 2022, and literally dumped everything we relocated from there into the rear garden and shed at this house, with Rod telling me he would sort it out in the next few months. But when he first got sick back in July of that same year, with what we now know was the start of his cancer, he wasn't strong enough to sort it out. I'm a person who likes to have a tidy house and garden. I dislike clutter and mess. Rod, on the other hand, is what I would describe as a hoarder. For him, he could see nothing wrong with half-finished projects. For me, as the months rolled on and here we were, in 2023, with full on cancer treatment, the mess in the back yard became a torture for me.

Rod's pride wouldn't let him ask for help, but for me it was completely de-motivating that we couldn't plan the work we wanted to do. My mood was getting heavier each day. I wanted to get contractors in, but Rod wanted me to wait. On reflection, I should have just over-ridden him and gone ahead. It would have given me something to look forward to, along with a sense of achievement, instead of half-finished jobs.

As the months rolled on, I gradually got used to the idea this was our life for now. I kept reminding myself it wouldn't be this way forever.

I started to look forward to Kate and Kev's posts, dreaming of the days when Rod and I could go there. It became a travel guide for me, I could look at all their pictures and the places they are visiting and decide, yes or no, if I wanted to visit them. I loved watching the faces of our granddaughters as they video called and told me all about their adventures.

The gypsy soul in me knows I still have time to do these things. Travel is in my blood and, if given the choice, I would roam this country from end to end. Perhaps this was just my way of escaping my current reality, fantasising about the day I could travel as a way of escape. Some might say it's running away, and yes, there's some truth in that. I did want to run away, I wanted our life to go back to normal, the normal we had before cancer, the one where we had lots of small trips plotted and long-term plans. The one where cancer was no longer part of our lives! There's a certain guilt that comes with that too, the shadow side of your soul, where you feel guilty for being jealous that other's lives are going ahead and yours is frozen in time.

I journaled much about this guilt and my feelings of life on hold, which certainly helped me to process my emotions and bring me to a place of living our lives alongside cancer. There was no going back to pre-cancer days, so somehow we had to integrate Rod's diagnosis into our everyday lives and make new contracts with ourselves, new soul plans.

Armed with this new understanding of myself, I started to make plans for small trips with Rod. Sometimes it was just a day trip to somewhere I've not been before. We took our caravan to his brother's property three hours away, just for the weekend, which felt like a mini holiday. We began achieving small things, tidying up, de-cluttering, shopping days together again, and with Rod progressing to monthly chemo and his body holding up well, it gave us even more opportunity to travel and start planning again.

Life felt like it had started moving forward.

MY DARKEST DAYS

In the beginning there was so much to do, so many appointments to attend, that I didn't really have time to pause and think about how I was really doing. Yes, I was journaling and doing self-reflection, but I was still running on high stress levels which we know to be the fight, flight, or freeze response, and I was very much in fight or flight. When we got to the stage of Rod's cancer being asleep and we went to monthly chemotherapy treatments, life started to stabilise, but my mental health took a battering.

It was at this point that dark thoughts began to creep in. I started thinking what the point of being here was, if this is what the Universe has planned for us? Who would miss me, with everyone else getting on with life? Everything felt hopeless. Now, remember, I am trained in supporting clients through suicide ideation but never once thought I would be that person. I started to recognise the path I was headed down and reached out to my friend, Jodi, who was also a counsellor. We talked things through, and I acknowledged that it was purely ideation at this stage, and I had no plans to take my life. I knew, deep down, that I needed to be here for Rod, for myself, for Kate, the girls, and my family.

I hold such strong beliefs in the power of the mind that I convinced myself I didn't need medication, but one day I found myself sitting in my car outside a shop, and I started to cry and couldn't stop. I sat there for two hours crying, unable to drive anywhere. Finally, I messaged Jodi and told her what was going on, where I was, and she messaged me the name of a doctor to talk to. I rang and made the appointment to see her. This level of situational depression confused me. This was not me; how could I be that person? I didn't recognise these feelings, nor did I know how to deal with them.

I was also, at this point, feeling very angry with myself for not feeling in control of my mental health. I feel so passionately about the power of the mind that when I couldn't control the thoughts I was having, I became very hard on myself.

When the doctor told me I was severely depressed, she recommended medication. I agreed to give them a try and returned home. It was difficult telling Rod and Kate how I was feeling. I felt selfish because he was fighting so hard to live, and I just wanted to return to the spirit world and not be here. Kate told me how proud she was of me for taking the first step, acknowledging how I was feeling and reaching out for help. I found that ironic considering I was normally the one telling others this.

We had a three-week holiday planned, in between the monthly chemotherapy sessions, with our friends, Matt and Kay, and their children, Noah and Indi, and I told myself I would start the tablets then. I kept putting off taking them, telling myself I would take them tomorrow, and often talking over with Kay during those three weeks, how I was feeling about taking them or not taking them. I kept saying I would take them, but something wasn't sitting right with me. That intuitive feeling that I could get through this without the use of medication was getting stronger. I meditate daily, write in my journal and tune into my higher self regularly. The more I reflected and asked for guidance on how I got to this dark place, the clearer it became. I started to talk to myself about my feelings, the way I would a client. I recognised that my body had been in trauma response for so many months now, that when it started to stabilise, my body was fighting hard to stay in fight or flight mode, which at the time felt safer. This high level of stress was my new normal and I was unable to regulate my nervous system.

I recognised that I needed to replace this stress with something else, so I began to change my focus to planning our future, planning short trips and what I could de-clutter from my life. This planning was not intended to be a way of keeping my body busy, but to help my body remember what *calm* and *daily life* feel like. I am a firm believer that we hold stress not just in our brains but also in our bodies, and when we release the stress from the body, it frees up the mind to start to think more clearly and calmly. Kay also encouraged me to step outside of my comfort zone and do things in those three weeks we were away that I wouldn't normally do. One of the things I remember was joining her at sunrise on the beach and diving into the freezing cold water, staying there for over 10 minutes. This was helpful in resetting my body. The more I reflected, the faster I got back to emotional regulation, my depression lifted, and my coping mechanisms grew stronger as did my return to my spiritual beliefs.

During this time, I also had a conversation with my good friend, Vicki. When I told her that I would wake up every morning with the thought *my husband has cancer*, she suggested I finish that sentence with *and he is getting treatment for it*. It was a great suggestion, and now when I wake up with this thought I tell myself, *my husband has cancer and he's having treatment for it*. When I think and say it that way, it leaves me feeling so much calmer and optimistic about the future.

I returned to the doctor after three weeks away and we redid the test. My depression level was down to only mild, without taking medication. I am in awe of how much power the mind has over our lives, and just as incredible is the mind and body connection. To release trauma from the body it's important to look at where the energy is blocked, and find ways that work for you. For me, and many of my clients, we have found that movement is the key. I would recommend that anyone feeling stuck, depressed, or having dark thoughts, should get up and move. Stretch, dance, walk, run - anything you can do to support the body in releasing trauma.

Rod and I started watching happy movies, laughing at comedies, looking for something to be grateful for in each day. Look around in nature and appreciate flowers or even the colour of the trees - small moments of joy, acknowledging where we are now in this moment without letting the fear of the future overcome us.

I think it's important to mention though, that whilst I was able to pull myself out of the dark place I was in, I did so through many years of specialist training in my profession. I acknowledge and recognise that this doesn't always work for others, so there is absolutely nothing wrong with taking medication on a doctor's advice and I am a big advocate for this when other alternatives are not working. I believe that there needs to be a rounded holistic approach to mental health, utilising both medical and complimentary therapies, individualised to what works for each person.

THE JOURNEY

Some people I've observed don't like the saying "a cancer journey", but for me it IS a journey. It's a journey of self-discovery. There are so many things I'm learning about myself, about Rod, and our relationship that I didn't know before.

Cancer is an unknown. When they tell us it's sleeping, we are left in limbo. Tim (oncologist) feels it will wake up again, but the unknown is when or if. What our destination will be is still unclear. We all must face death at some stage, that's one thing we know for sure about the human life cycle. So, for us, what does the journey mean? How can we make this journey easier to cope with? Do we live our lives in fear or do we go on as normal, making normal plans, normal financial decisions. These are all questions I reflected on constantly.

At one of Rod's chemotherapy sessions I sat and observed a woman who was also there having treatment. She was crying and continued to cry the whole time we were there. My heart was very heavy for her, for her struggle and for her partner sitting next to her, watching her pain and sadness. Rod, on the other hand was cheerful, being cheeky and having a laugh with the chemo nurses. This made me more curious about the journey. Rod's diagnosis is one that is classified as advanced and incurable. I had no idea what the diagnosis was for this woman in the chemo suite that day, but it showed me the difference between two people's individual journey. Do we have to make it a struggle? Both will have the same destination, one might be faster than the other, but I believe it's the power of the mind that separates us from each other when dealing with trauma like this.

Some days the road on this journey seems straight forward even though it's a little narrow, others it feels like it's winding back on itself or covered with mountains to climb. There are many forks in the road with choices to be made. Often, we have no idea whether we have made the right choice, but we are too far down the road to turn back.

When it comes to your partner, it's natural that we want to protect them and make their journey easier, but one thing I've learnt is that I can't control that; I only have control over my part of this journey and remember to honour my feelings as I go. For me, I've come to release the struggle and surrendered it up to the Universe, and I chose to go with the flow of living completely in this moment.

I document my journey daily and when I read it back, I am often surprised at how far I have come. How much stronger I feel now than those first few months and weeks. I document this process by taking a few deep breaths to settle my nervous system, and I lean into how I am feeling about this journey right now and then let the words flow through free writing.

MY ANGER AT ROD

Anger is not something that occurs often in our relationship. I would say frustration with each other is more our style. But when Rod kept working, even though it was from home, I was very angry. He had so much personal leave owing to him and yet he wasn't taking it. I had shelved my own business to focus on supporting him, his treatment and spending time together. When he chose not to do the same and keep working, I really lost my temper.

Now, I know this is my issue to deal with, but I spiraled into feeling he didn't care about me enough to take his leave. He didn't value our dream of travelling and living life the best we could, as much as me. His work is more important than me. Either he was in complete denial, or he didn't love me, and I chose to go the "he didn't love me" road. My level of anger was building every day that I saw him sitting at his computer, working away as though nothing had changed. I felt like he would still be sitting there until he was too ill to do so, and that he was cheating me out of the quality time we have left together. Every time I looked at his computer screen, I wanted to smash it, feeling that I was in a three-way relationship - me, Rod, and his work. I know this might sound extremely harsh and irrational, but when trauma strikes your life, you don't think rationally until you have time to process and work through the shock and what this means for you and your life.

I started lashing out at him, and then would feel guilty for doing so. Thinking to myself, *he has cancer for gawd's sake, who am I to be so needy right now?* I had been wanting Rod to retire for a few years, but he kept putting it off, saying maybe one more year. Now he has cancer and our hopes and dreams of travelling in retirement had gone out the window, or so I thought. I felt cheated and betrayed. I remember telling a friend that I didn't want to be standing by his grave site feeling resentful, when I should be grieving him.

Many of his family, friends, and colleagues, all with good intentions, were saying to me that work is giving him something to focus on, to take his mind off things, to keep him going. But in my shoes, work was stealing our precious time together and they were being completely insensitive to me. I know this was not their intention, but in their efforts to support Rod, my feelings got overlooked, which made it worse, and I took it out on Rod.

It took many conversations, and a few spears thrown at each other, to come to a compromise. I also had to do a lot of deep reflection. Who was I truly angry at? I realised it was me, for investing all my time and energy into planning a future that, at the time, I felt was out of reach... for putting my dreams on hold for so many years whilst he chose when to retire... for linking my own happiness to Rod and not being strong enough to do things without him. I know I could have travelled without him, but I didn't want to, I wanted to share that journey with him. I kept telling myself back then, before the cancer diagnosis, that he will retire next year and we will travel then. But life had a different plan for Rod, one that I couldn't control.

I have a belief that the Universe has a way of slowing you down, giving you subtle messages and when you don't listen to those messages they get stronger and harder. I felt that Rod hadn't listened to these messages until the Universe intervened in a huge way.

I wanted him to give up work, and yet here he was still holding onto it. I said many hurtful things to him, like the time I told him 'work would replace him in a heartbeat after he's gone, but his family and friends couldn't.' I was angry at him for getting sick, for not listening to the Universe, not looking after his health better, for pushing himself to work harder, even though deep down, I knew this was unfair to him. My anger also brought up feelings of guilt and shame for feeling this way.

Eventually, as everyone started to understand just how serious his diagnosis was, they also started to understand what I was feeling, and asked him 'why not give up work and make the most of his life now?' Financial issues were not a concern as we both knew we were in a good place financially, so why was he holding on so tightly?

Even though Rod is open to holistic therapies, he put his whole treatment in Tim's hands. I wanted him to try new things, change his lifestyle completely, but he was reluctant. This frustrated me even more. In my mind I was thinking if this was me, I would be doing everything possible. But it wasn't my life, it was his. I wanted him to talk to me, let me in with his thoughts and emotions. Rod is very much a closed book and finds it so hard to communicate. I find this aspect of him extremely frustrating, not only as his wife but also as a counsellor. Whenever I ask him an open-ended question he will answer in the third person, removing himself from the emotion. An example of this was when I asked him how he was feeling about the diagnosis, and he replied, "Well no one wants cancer, do they?". My response was something like 'that's not what I asked and I'm not talking about no one, I'm asking you.' Having Rod open up is what I equate to pulling teeth, you really have to dig deep with him.

Through my frustration and anger I started nagging and pushing him, and the more I pushed, the more he dug in and shut down. I got a glimpse into how relationships can break down after a cancer diagnosis due to the different viewpoints. I wasn't going to let that happen to us, we were not going to be that couple. My relationship counselling training would certainly stretch me through this journey.

I realised that something had to give, that this shouldn't be a battle or power struggle between us. This was my issue and I had to let it go, to try and understand this from his perspective whilst still holding onto my own future dreams. I started to plan things in my day for me to do, to separate myself from him and step back into my own identity. The less focused I became on him working, the more he released his grip on it.

We made a compromise that in between the chemo sessions we would take short trips and he could balance that by continuing to support his work colleagues. I know how much Rod loves me, and whilst I don't need his love to feel worthy, I do recognise that my happiness is my responsibility. I made the choice to stop working based on my own feelings, and I understand I can't expect him to do the same. To date, it's still a transition in progress, but my anger has faded and my positive outlook to life has increased.

SUPPORT NETWORKS

One thing I was told right from the start was to find a supportive network and to not be afraid to reach out to people for help. As a counsellor, I know all too well how powerful and therapeutic talking to others, and even group work, can be. Sharing your journey with others who are experiencing similar situations helps you feel less alone and isolated. I would encourage anyone going through this journey to find a good support group.

There are downsides however, being in too many groups can be draining and take up a lot of time. When Rod was first diagnosed, I went into overdrive joining groups ; searching for information, looking for success stories, and wanting to connect with others. Reading all the posts, and feeling like I should comment to give support to others became exhausting. The counsellor in me wanted to help others, but in that moment, I only had enough emotional capacity to support myself, Rod, and our family. I started to scale back on the groups I was in, and stayed active in only one or two where I felt I could contribute and not become exhausted.

The other downside with being in too many cancer groups is that members die, or their family members die. Every time I read a post about someone losing their loved one it was a trigger and sad reminder that I might lose Rod to this disease. This allowed the fear to creep back in and my energy vibration to become low. I had to keep reminding myself that everyone's circumstances and journeys are different, and this didn't necessarily mean that Rod was going to die.

One of the hardest losses was a young woman from the UK, only 29 years of age, with whom I used to communicate regularly. She was diagnosed at the same time as Rod with the same rare primary cardiac angiosarcoma. We followed each other's journey closely, offering support and celebrating small wins and successes. I remember how excited but fearful she was when she was told that she was eligible to have surgery to remove the tumour. This is something that Rod so desperately wanted himself, as I'm sure a lot of others in our group also want. The thought being, if the tumour is removed before it has metastasized, it gives hope to a cure or at least a longer life. But when she developed complications after surgery, I and others in the group became very worried. We were anxiously looking for her posts. I was sending her messages with no response. Then the message finally came from another in our group, who was close to the family, that a few days before, in October 2023, and after a short battle, she had passed away. As I am writing this, I still get emotional when I think of her. I couldn't believe it, I was in shock, how could she be gone, only 10 months after diagnosis. When I told Rod, the look on his face was heartbreaking. I could see that he was crushed, that this operation was supposed to save her life, not take it. We were heartbroken for her, her family and for our group. It was a sad reminder of how cruel this disease can be. We reflected on it a few days later, that maybe it was a good thing that Rod hadn't had the surgery.

Finding a support team that you can lean on when you need to is crucial. I am fortunate that I have a solid network of family and friends as does Rod. Rod's brothers are the ones he turns to first, along with a few close friends who come and have a beer or cup of tea with him, often dropping in fillets of his favourite fish or a crayfish, joking and laughing and generally making his situation feel so much lighter. We have one friend, Troy, who used to come and mow the lawn for us, his way of showing support for which we were extremely grateful. And Colin and Ann visit most Sundays, sometimes for a cup of tea, other times for a drink. Their visits, and the fact that we don't talk about Rod's cancer, make our world feel just that little bit more normal.

We were so blessed that Murray, who is Rod's manager at work, is one of the most supportive people we know. He immediately took the pressure off Rod, diverting some of his work to others, whilst at the same time encouraging Rod to only do as much he felt like. Knowing the balance between Rod still having a purpose, and yet taking the time to rest and recuperate through the treatment cycles, was important. This meant that Rod could work from home and not have to be on site, where we recognised he would be at risk of overtiring himself and possibly picking up an infection.

Most of my friends are all either in the counselling, support or holistic field like me, so I find it easy to reach out, and do so in different ways. My family are amazing and check in with me regularly to see how I'm doing. I know I wouldn't be able to face this journey without them, but there are some things I find I can't tell them; some of my thoughts I know they wouldn't understand.

When I was looking for support groups my go-to initially was through social media pages. There are so many different groups available and often ones for a particular type of cancer. I preferred ones that were a private group so that we could talk openly, without others attached to my social media pages seeing what I was asking or commenting on.

Other places I researched were within my local community and the cancer council where I live. I also sought out a colleague of mine trained in grief counselling, and asked her if she would take me on as a client (yes, counsellors need counselling too). It really helped me to work through my thoughts, fears and emotions with someone who wasn't directly involved in our day-to-day lives. I am a big advocate of finding someone outside of your normal circle so you can share, explore and just feel heard with.

MOVING THROUGH FEAR

There are many types of fear when it comes to cancer: fear of a loved one dying or being in pain; fear of the treatment, side effects and whether it will work; fear of what this will mean for us; fear of telling children, family, and friends.

Then there are other fears. How will I cope financially, on my own? I fear living by myself, growing old without my partner. What if I'm not able to cope?

Initially, all those fears crept in. The fear of the unknown was the worst. Not being able to see into the future nor control it, was terrifying. I kept playing over and over in my mind scenes of me in the future, a future without Rod. Worried about finances, even though this is not really an issue. I worried about where I would live as I didn't think I would want to stay in this house without him. The fear of him dying was excruciating. Every moment of every day, I felt fear creep in. Every little cough or groan from him sent me into panic, thinking it's the cancer. I became obsessed with asking him, over and over, how he was feeling.

I had thoughts of *I'm only 61 years of age... if Rod dies I most likely will still have twenty plus years left to live on my own. It's going to be a lonely twenty plus years.* I could never imagine myself with anyone else. Rod and I are a good team and the thought of doing life without him was painful.

There is also the fear every time Rod is due for a PET scan. We call this scanxiety, and it triggers all those other fears to surface again. Scanxiety is a term I have now come to terms with. Even through all our positive mindset, the weeks leading up to the next scan, which for Rod is every three months, my mind starts to wander. What if it's woken up again, what if it's spread, what if the treatment has stopped working? All of these are normal fears and I take the time to tune into them, one by one. I usually take some deep breaths and ask myself, *what if it hasn't woken up? What if it hasn't spread? What if the treatment is still working?* I remind myself that the treatment is working so far, Rod looks well and is functioning well, so why would I allow this worry to overshadow what we have right in this moment? I try to put the scan to the back of my mind or not focus on it all day. Distraction is vital here.

I also had the fear of going out, socialising, travelling, attending events. His immune system had taken a battering with the chemotherapy, and what if he gets an infection? There was a moment I remember when we went out to a local hotel for a drink and some dinner. Because Rod hadn't been seen much over those few months, there were a number of people there who we knew, and they all wanted to come over to our table and visit. I'm not great around people who have had too much to drink at the best of times, so when people came over, knowing that they had a bit to drink, I felt myself starting to withdraw and shrink away from them. I got very concerned they were too close to Rod, angry at myself that we weren't wearing masks. One person was so close I thought he was going to kiss Rod. I was horrified, and the more people came over the more panicked I became. What if they had Covid, what if they had a cold, what if they had gastro. All these fears running through my head. In the end, my overwhelm got too much and I said to Rod, "We need to get you out of here."

All these fears are real and need to be addressed. But one thing I've learnt is that fear is your body's way of trying to keep you safe, but it also robs you of many moments of joy and happiness. When I live my life through a fear-based lens, I miss out on the good things that are happening in the here and now. Yes, there is a real possibility of losing Rod, but right now he's still here, and we can still laugh and love each other, share intimacy, and do things together. I refuse to let fear hold me back from what is good in my life right now. All we have is right now in this very moment, so why waste it with the energy of fear?

It doesn't mean I have to stop reflecting on what the future holds for us and for me. But I no longer allow myself to sit in that space for too long. I remember thinking back to when we had our old dog, Rainey, who had to be euthanised. On her last day we gave her everything she loved. She ate chocolate, a hamburger, we took her to the beach and gave her a day filled with love and joy. She probably lived her best life in that one day. We stayed with her until she took her last breath. Did she know it was going to be her last day? Probably not. Would she have been any different if she had? Probably not. That got me thinking that dogs live completely in the moment, so why not humans?

We can choose to live our lives consumed by fear or we can choose to make the most of every day. I'm choosing the latter. I look for moments of gratitude in each day. Each smile I get from Rod, each touch of the hand reminds me what we have right now. We plan, a future with him still in it. After all, the future is a mere second from now. I hold strong spiritual beliefs that we never truly lose someone. They just step out of our line of sight. Energetically, we are still connected to those we love and can still communicate with them, just in a way that seems out of the ordinary physical reality.

The future will come, no matter how much we try and avoid it. We can make it as much a struggle, as we can enjoyable. We each get to choose how we want it to be. My tip is to address each fear as they arise and try to alleviate this in a way that will work for you such as I did in the paragraphs above. Look to challenge those fears. I believe in the power of positive mindset and its ability to heal the body, and I remind myself that not every day has to be a sad one, which is why I actively pursue happy moments so that every day is not one consumed by Rod's cancer diagnosis.

BODY CHANGES & SEXUAL INTIMACY

I wanted to include this subject because it's not often talked about. Whilst this is a very personal subject, Rod and I talked over how much to share with you. I promised myself that I wouldn't sugarcoat anything and want to be completely open about this journey. So, let's dive in. If the subject of sex makes you feel uncomfortable, you might want to skip this chapter. Additionally, if any of our family and friends are reading this book, please skip this chapter, or if you choose to read it, promise me you will never mention it to me.

When Rod was first diagnosed with a suspicious mass, we were in shock and disbelief. I wanted to physically be as close to him as possible, wanting to hold his hand, needing to hug him, having him close by. But I was frightened of having sex. I was worried it would put more pressure on his heart or that it would hurt him. Our first time being intimate after hearing the news, I cried all the way through. All I kept thinking was how much I loved the feel of his skin and his unique smell, and if I lost him I would miss this so much. I felt guilty for crying, wondering what Rod must have thought. And I say this with a smile on my face, that Rod being Rod wanted to carry on with our sex life as normal.

For me though, the stress and trauma we were going through weighed heavily on my mind, which then affected my libido. I didn't feel like having sex, but if I said no, Rod might feel like I didn't want him anymore because of his cancer. The last thing I wanted him to feel was that he wasn't whole, attractive, or loved. It was very difficult to have those conversations, so in his best interests we continued to have sex.

Each time we did, I felt heavy, and I kept thinking about the monster growing inside him. It felt like it was taunting me, telling me it had control and was going to take him away from me. That might sound weird to some, but I believe we are all things energy, and this was just a piece of dark energy that needed to go. It was like a battle between us, the tumour and me. By having sex with my husband, I was sending it a strong message that I still held the balance of power over his heart.

When it came to treatment time and chemotherapy was about to start, we began researching the side effects. One site mentioned it could cause a lack of libido. I remember laughing to myself as I was reading it, *Well you don't know my husband.* We also looked into whether he can have sex whilst undertaking treatment. The google rabbit hole was vague on this subject with not a lot of credible information out there. Both Rod and I felt too embarrassed to ask Tim, his oncologist, for advice about sex, so we kept researching ourselves. I was extremely wary of transmission of the chemotherapy drugs through bodily fluids. We knew that we had to be careful about the toilet, shower, not sharing cups, etcetera but were still unsure about sex.

Rod managed to find some information that recommended using condoms. Condoms!!! We had never used those in the entire time we had been together. Armed with this information he went and bought some after I refused to. I told him this is a small town, and I don't want to be seen buying condoms and having people talk about me. Sounds ridiculous now, but I wasn't prepared to go into a pharmacy or supermarket and sneakily try and purchase them. So off he went, and came home with a few different types and sizes. This was one of the funniest moments and I remember telling him, "You're being a bit ambitious, there's absolutely no way we are going to use that many."

Before we got the chance to use them, I found some information that suggested we wait seventy-two hours after treatment and then it should be safe to have unprotected sex. We decided to give that a try, even though Rod would try and convince me it had been seventy-two hours, when it hadn't.

Rod has been very fortunate to not experience too many side effects with his treatment, and the chemotherapy certainly hasn't affected his libido. For me, however, one of the things I didn't expect was the sudden changes to his body. Rod has a decent amount of body hair, and the granddaughters often called him a hairy monkey. When you are with someone for so many years, you become accustomed to every part of their body. What it feels like, looks like, how it smells. I love the fact that his body has hair, and I would often run my fingers through his chest hair. So, I was taken by surprise by how I felt when, within three weeks of treatment, Rod had lost all his hair all over his body.

I had prepared myself for him to lose it from his head and eyebrows, but it was a shock to see his body completely hairless. He looked like a different person completely. When we had sex, I struggled because it didn't feel like him. It felt alien and I couldn't find enjoyment. I just wanted my husband back. Of course, at the time I couldn't tell him this. I didn't want to hurt his feelings. The other thing I found was that losing his hair was a reminder of how ill his body was. A constant smack in the face - my husband has cancer.

Once again, I knew that I had to change my mindset around this. I began to focus on parts of his body that I found attractive. I would touch his smooth face, and marvel at how soft his skin felt. The scar on his chest from the biopsy was now very prominent, and I focused on how incredible the body is at healing itself. I started to find it interesting and fascinating how his body was changing through this process. He was still the same man, the one I love, and I looked past the exterior to remember that it is his soul that I find truly attractive. Our energy was again blending well.

When the treatment went from weekly to monthly, Rod's hair started to grow back. I was amazed at how quickly it grew. Suddenly there was a different person again in front of me. This one had a grey beard and hair. This hair was different, soft, almost like rabbit fur. The nurses in the chemo suite were as excited as we were, and they wanted to touch his head. We would laugh at this and the attention he was getting. I had never seen Rod with a beard before, and he had this sexy rugged look about him. I started calling him my Sean Connery. As it continued to grow, he was unsure how to trim a beard so eventually he decided to shave it off.

As his hair was growing back, it was doing so in an odd way. It was growing up to a point on his head, and we laughed about this often. It was like two waves meeting at the top of his head. I remember being in a restaurant, and as Rod went to the counter to order a guy standing next to him said "nice hair mate". Rod didn't tell him why it was like this, but we had a good laugh about it. I've found myself often looking at others who have been through chemo, with interest, noticing how their hair was growing back. I find it fascinating how the body adapts to changes. My nephew's wife, Sarah, now has curly hair after treatment and when I look at both her and Rod, I feel a sense of pride in their strength. Their hair is a testament to overcoming the harsh poison being injected into their bodies.

When I now look at Rod, with hair, I'm no longer reminded that he has cancer, but instead I see a man with a strong, positive mindset moving through this challenge with a sense of humour and resilience to adapt to any changes.

For me, it felt like in the space of five months I had been having sex with three different Rod's. Someone asked me which one I preferred, and I replied, "all of them". It was an interesting journey through my own emotions.

Needless to say, the condoms are still in the drawer unopened, and our sex life is intact, with a new level of intimacy that has us closer than ever.

SPIRITUAL BELIEFS & COMPLIMENTARY THERAPIES

When it comes to spiritual beliefs and spirituality, there are many images that come to mind. Every person has their own individual beliefs and ideas on this subject. Personally, I believe in a higher power, something greater than just myself. Some might call it God, Allah, Almighty Creator, Divinity, or the Universe. I like to use the words "the Universe". I believe in the Universe, my higher self, and our energetic connection to each other as coming from the same source. I believe in spirit guides and ancestors that can still communicate with us.

I was constantly searching for signs, seeking guidance from the Universe that everything was going to be okay. This might be a feather appearing at my feet, or a rainbow when I least expect it; all of which give me comfort. As a spiritual person, I often draw on my own intuition through the use of oracle cards, soul writing and meditation. Listening to the messages I'm being sent helps me to trust in what my soul needs for self-care, and how to move forward each day. I have a beautiful mentor, Marnie Cate, an extremely talented clairvoyant and spiritual teacher, who lives in Western Australia. It was in late June that I sat with Marnie for a reading, and we explored what the future held for me, and for us as a couple. I hadn't told Marnie about my idea of writing a book, but it wasn't long before the guides brought it up. We discussed it together and, in that moment, I knew that writing a book about our journey and my own emotions through this was something I needed to do, not just for others but also for myself as a way of processing my own trauma.

As a holistic therapist, I am trained in many modalities such as mainstream counselling, breathwork, somatic therapy, energy healing, sound healing and EFT (tapping). I use a combination of these in my own life, and with my clients. I have always believed that our own soul and the Universe have a plan for us. What I sometimes struggle with is why that plan might be such a traumatic one. Nonetheless, I have always managed to maintain a positive attitude to life.

So, when Rod was first diagnosed, I went into shock. My energy vibration was very low. I believe when your vibration is low it encourages stress and dis-ease to grow within your body. Unable to pull myself out of this state, I was getting headaches, tummy upsets and a few other minor health issues. I started to question my spiritual beliefs and stopped doing my daily practice. I was spiraling, becoming increasingly negative and judgmental. This was someone I didn't recognise. The shadow side of me stepped out from behind that pillar and into the spotlight. I did as I always do, a great deal of reflection and journaling. I wrote about being angry at the Universe and no longer wanted to communicate with my spirit guides, ignoring signs from spirit. I distrusted my own higher self and my intuition, feeling completely disconnected and lost. I recognised this was just part of the process I needed to work through. In fact, I have drifted back and forth a few times in this journey, which I write about in my reflection of my darkest days.

When it comes to energy therapists, I want to point out that it is not the person facilitating the energy work who holds any form of healing power. They are merely a conduit to bring forward the right energetic conditions to allow healing to occur, whether that be a healing of the nervous system, or the mind. My personal thoughts on cancer are such that it isn't just something you get, unless it is caused by an environmental change like asbestos or sun damage. It's a cellular change in your body, that something triggered to create the right conditions for the cancer to grow. I believe that if your body can create it, then it can heal it, and that healing can take many forms. I am not in any way advocating away from conventional treatments, because I am certainly not qualified or knowledgeable enough to make that call. What I am advocating for is an integrated approach to be undertaken. Part of that integrated approach includes energy therapy, mindset, breathwork, meditation, and when necessary, medical intervention. Believing in the power of the body to heal itself is just as important as putting your life in the hands of good health professionals and we're fortunate that Rod is in very good hands with Tim, his oncologist, and the medical team at the cancer centre.

Once we knew what we were dealing with, I asked Rod if he would like to get on the healing table. I'm grateful that Rod is open to most of my suggestions and has been on the healing table before, along with having a few sound healing sessions with me. What I wasn't prepared for was once he was on the table, I could feel the heaviness of the tumour's energy. As I started to undertake the work on him through Reiki, it felt like it was getting angrier with me. I kept focusing on, that it had no place to be there in his body and that it needed to go. I had a moment where I felt something shift in his body and release its hold. It was in that moment I knew that love would always be stronger than evil. In the meantime, while I was having this battle, Rod was on the table relaxed and resting, completely oblivious to the struggle going on.

I've had Rod back on the table a few times since then and notice a difference in both his energy and that of the tumour. As we lie in bed at night, I ask for healing to occur to cleanse his body of the cancer cells. It was at his next PET scan that we got the news that the tumour was shrinking, the chemotherapy had put it to sleep, and it hadn't spread any further. When I had time to reflect on this news, I thanked the Universe for providing the right energetic conditions for healing to occur, through the power of Rod's own beliefs and the conventional medical treatment he was undertaking.

But please know that, once again, I am not saying that Reiki or energy healing is a cure, but I do believe it helps to support the body by regulating the nervous system to relax, which in turn allows healing to occur on a cellular level. This, coupled with conventional treatment, provided us with the right conditions to fight this monster. My faith in the Universe and my spiritual connection to my own self was restored.

I talk a lot about creating the right energetic conditions for healing to occur, which flows through into the environment and the people you surround yourself with. If your external environment is noisy, messy, and filled with stress, then I believe these are not the right energetic conditions. At home, I try to create a calm and soft environment for Rod. I light candles, diffuse essential oils, have soft lamps in the house including salt lamps, and I play calm music. Rod regularly has magnesium baths to help relax him and ease the side effects from the chemotherapy, and when we are watching the television in the evening, the lights are down low, the house is in a calm state and even the shows we watch are uplifting and relatively calm. We eat well, a variety of fresh fruit and vegetables coupled with healthy proteins, and prepare all our meals at home. I believe this environment is helping to support his healing.

As most do, when someone is diagnosed with cancer, we go down the google rabbit hole seeking any research and information we can find to support the body, and look for a cure. I was no different. I spent a great deal of time down that rabbit hole. I was researching conventional treatment along with holistic and alternative treatments. I came across some interesting articles and a little bit of research on the use of turkey tail mushrooms as an immune support for someone with cancer. When I nervously broached this with Tim, he shot me down immediately, telling me the research wasn't conclusive and that scientific trials in the laboratory doesn't necessarily mean it will work on humans. He told me that I could get stuck down that rabbit hole, wasting much of my time and energy.

I knew what he was saying as I had been down that rabbit hole a great deal, and agreed to let the subject drop, for the time being. I later spoke about this with Rod and acknowledged that because there was no set protocol for treating his rare cancer, from a scientific point of view, if I added something to the mix of the conventional treatment, how would we really know what was working? Was it the chemotherapy drugs or the turkey tail mushrooms? I agreed not to use it until we got to the point of the cancer being asleep, then I would look at it again, purely through the lens of supporting his immune system. In the meantime, a member of one of the support groups I am in mentioned that her oncologist, a top physician in the US who specialises with angiosarcoma, had indicated it wouldn't hurt to give turkey tail mushrooms a try.

As I write this book, Rod has now been having turkey tail mushroom extract occasionally, with only the minimum dosage required and I believe it has given him more energy, even if it is a placebo effect. It will be interesting to watch in the future as further studies are made on natural therapies and the effect on cancer cells. I also look for anti-inflammatory foods, herbs and spices that we can use in our cooking to help support him but am careful to check with his medical team first, and I would also encourage anyone to speak with their medical team before trying any alternative therapies or medication to make sure there are no contraindications.

My thoughts of death and dying are something I talk about often. I believe that the soul goes on, and although the physical body may be gone from this earth, the soul is still present and we can communicate with it whenever we want to. Death itself is not something that scares me, it is a natural process within the cycle of life, and I believe when we die, we return to source, which is a place of pure love.

Am I scared of losing someone? Yes, because that human part of my soul knows what that pain feels like. Losing someone you love is painful and sad, but remembering that the soul lives on can give much comfort through this period of mourning and grieving. Whilst it is hard to talk about death and dying with loved ones who are ill or nearing end of life, it can also be a moment of deep connection and comfort.

I've often asked Rod, what his thoughts are when it comes to dying and what he believes happens to the soul and the body. I believe that talking about the unknown and exploring our personal views also removes the fear and stigma. In other cultures around the world, talking about death and dying is not viewed as something taboo and they embrace the whole ceremony of life. It provides the opportunity to share memories, to honour and witness those final moments with love and gratitude for sharing lives together. I've often thought that when my time comes, I hope I am surrounded by those I love, and that it's a sacred moment and not one filled with fear.

OUR FIRST HOLIDAY

Monthly chemo has made it possible for us to dip our toes in the water and start to travel. In July 2023 we were very excited to plan our first holiday away since September 2022. We were taking our caravan to Shark Bay in Western Australia, 1000 km north of where we currently live. When we started talking about it, our friends, Matt and Kay, with their two children, Noah and Indi, said they would love to join us. I felt comforted by this, I was a little nervous at travelling so far away from home, especially from the hospital and Rod's oncologist. Rod has a small boat that goes on the roof of our car. In Australia we call them a tinny. Fishing and being in the boat are among Rod's favourite pastimes. He loves being in and on the water, and Shark Bay is an ideal place to take the boat.

I knew it was going to be a journey travelling that far, but we talked it over and decided we would only travel 300 to 400 kms each day and take a few days to get there and back. In the past it would have been normal for Rod and me to travel 700 plus kms a day towing the caravan, but this was a whole new reality. When we approached the subject of travel with Rod's oncologist, Tim, he was very supportive of the idea. He encourages Rod to do the things he loves and live his best life. Occasionally, he would give Rod an injection after his monthly chemo to help boost his immune system. The only downside to this treatment was intense bone pain as a side effect, however, being so far away from the hospital, it was going to be necessary for him to have one for this trip.

I started planning the trip, carefully mapping out places to stay that were nearby to medical facilities if we needed them. One of the risks for Rod with cardiac angiosarcoma is that part of the dead tissue from the tumour may break away and cause a stroke or heart attack. This is something that plays on my mind. Additionally, the week after chemo is when his immune system drops the most and we must be careful of infection, so we avoid crowded places. There is a lot to consider when travelling. So many medications to pack, masks, hand sanitiser, and even though it's our own caravan it must be cleaned more thoroughly and more frequently. Packing the car and caravan was exhausting, and we took our time to get it done. The day to leave had finally arrived. It almost felt euphoric, I never thought that six months earlier we would be going anywhere, let alone with our much-loved caravan and boat.

We arrived in Shark Bay and were extremely grateful to Matt and Kay who helped us set up quickly. Rod was tired but happy. It took him a couple of days to get the boat off the roof and get his energy up to fish. We travel with our two dogs, so I stayed behind with them at the caravan park while they all went out fishing. Kay went out with Rod in his boat that first day and thank goodness she did. The chemo side effects had taken its toll on Rod's fingernails and toenails. They were lifting, coming off, bleeding and very painful. Kay was baiting all his hooks and pulling the crab pots for him.

Being on holiday in his boat and the warmer weather certainly improved both our moods, and our souls felt happy for the first time in ages. My brother Steve, his wife Tracey, and my niece Jen, with her daughter Isabelle, and Jen's partner Jacob, came up to join us for a few days. This was so good for me, being in a different setting and away from all the sadness we had gone through, spending time with them really made it even more special. We had three wonderful weeks away and our nerves about travelling were abated. We decided that if all went well and the cancer was still asleep after the next scan, we would definitely do more.

I remember sitting one day on the beach, just silently watching, reflecting, and grateful for the time we were spending there. Dolphins slowly making their way past, and I wrote this in my journal.

> I sit here listening to the crashing waves. Watching a pod of dolphins swim past. People are slowly starting to wake up and go about their daily lives. All travellers - just like us. Each with their own traumas. No one is immune to trauma. We integrate it into our lives and tell each other our stories. How many people have sat where I am sitting now, I wonder. Staring out at the ocean, wondering what lies ahead. How many will sit here long after I'm gone. Yet the ocean still ebbs and flows. It's tides turning, flowing back and forth, watching me watching it. There's a comfort in knowing that its life is never ending and that it will continue to bring peace to others as it does me in this moment.

Rod's next PET scan was scheduled for the week after we returned. We had discussed selling our old caravan and buying a new, a slightly smaller one that would be easier for us to manage. We thought we would get pushback from our family and friends, wondering why we would spend all that money when Rod's future was so uncertain, but to our surprise they were all very supportive. They all know how important it is to have a plan for the future, something to look forward to.

We talked long and hard about it, and eventually decided that if the cancer was still sleeping, we would do it, honouring our commitment to each other to live completely in this moment. Needless to say, we were elated when his scan showed it still asleep, the spots on his lungs no longer detectable, and the original heart tumour had shrunk even more. Two days later we bought our new caravan and excitedly began planning another trip away.

One of the things I've learnt through my google rabbit hole research, indicates that stress may be a contributing factor to cancer waking up again. So, for us, the trips away are enjoyable and provide Rod with the right environment to heal and rest. We feel so much more confident that this can now be achieved.

ROD'S PERSPECTIVE

I had been thinking a great deal on the fact that this book, even though it reflects both our journeys, is written purely from my own perspective with not much input from Rod. We had talked about what we wanted to achieve by writing it and who we hoped it might support.

I've mentioned before that Rod is an internaliser and finds it hard to express his thoughts, so I talked it over with him and suggested that whilst we were travelling across the Nullabor on our three-month trip away, I would like to do an interview with him. I told him I thought it would be helpful for others reading this book to hear it from his perspective. Whilst we didn't want him to relive the trauma, I felt that talking about it to me in that format might help him verbalise and process it himself. I was surprised when he agreed. The following conversation is a transcript of that interview:

Christine: Those first few days and weeks, what was it like for you, hearing those words - there's a suspicious mass.

Rod: When I first heard it, I was still groggy from the anesthetic, but when I realised that there was a mass there, I wasn't sure what it was. Lots of people initially were thinking about mesothelioma because of my work history and losing Mouse, who has always worked in the same place as me. I was fairly confident it wasn't mesothelioma, but you just don't know. [Mouse was Rod's work colleague and friend.]

Christine: Why were you so confident it wasn't mesothelioma?

Rod: Because I've always been fairly careful with safety and taking precautions in that area, so I didn't think it was.

Christine: What was going through your mind though?

Rod: Well, obviously hoping it wasn't, and that it was a non-cancerous tumour, so you hold onto the hope that it wasn't mesothelioma, and that the non-cancerous tumour could be removed.

Christine: Were you afraid of dying?

Rod: I didn't think about dying.

Christine: So you thought that whatever it is can be fixed?

Rod: Yes

Christine: What about when they said it's suspicious and it looked like it was cancerous?

Rod: Even though they indicated that they thought it was cancer, I was still under the belief that if it was removed, we would get rid of the cancer and move on with life.

Christine: What was it like seeing me cry all the time when we were first told?

Rod: Umm, it was very upsetting with the way you were dealing with it. You obviously thought it was worse than I did, and I guess there wasn't much I could do. I think it's your way of dealing with it and I left it like that. You would have a bit of a cry, and other times we would have a bit of a laugh, but I think it was just a natural way of expressing how you were feeling.

Christine: So those first few days and weeks after we found out it was suspicious, that it was most likely cancer, what were those days and weeks like for you? They seemed to drag on for me, but how did you experience it?

Rod: Well, you just want to have the test to find out, but I think the amount of time it took to finally get a sample and clearly say that it was cardiac angiosarcoma, even though they indicated that they had a fair idea themselves what it was and wouldn't say, was the most difficult. I think it dragged on a lot longer than we thought it would. That part was difficult, the waiting especially as, it was Christmas, with lots of specialists not available. Some of the specialists they wanted to talk to were away on holidays, and we had to wait because they wanted to do the first biopsy through my neck. And the specialist who needed to do that wasn't around so we waited longer than we probably should have. When we finally had that biopsy and then found out that they didn't get enough tissue to diagnose, it felt like we had gone through that process for nothing. Then we were back to waiting for the next step. I found that very hard.

Christine: Did it feel like we were going one step forward, two steps back?

Rod: Definitely.

Christine: Did you wonder at times what our family and friends were thinking, what was going through their minds? Were you concerned about their reactions?

Rod: Yes, I think everyone was the same, trying to find out what it was and how we were going to deal with it, whether it could be fixed and how it could be fixed. Trying to communicate with the rest of our family and friends when, at that time, we didn't know what to say to them because we didn't know ourselves. It was frustrating for them to ask, and we couldn't give them an answer except 'we have to have another test'... then another test and we still don't know. Whether or not they thought that we did know and weren't really telling them, I'm not sure. It came across that way from some of them, but as you know, we really didn't know. It was hard to communicate that to anyone.

Christine: Did you wonder about work at that point, what was going to happen or what was going to happen in the future? Did you have any thoughts at all about the future?

Rod: Well, you think about it but at that time we didn't know what we were dealing with, and I guess I was lucky enough to have an understanding manager in Murray, who as far as work goes, told me to focus on me and my health and not worry about work. I did that and I switched off from work.

Christine: Did you feel guilty about not being at work and letting the team down?

Rod: No, not really. At the time I was feeling fairly well, and unsure of what the outcome was going to be. I think, because we had been going through Covid and working from home, it didn't feel like it was a big deal, we could still stay in contact through the phone and video meetings. We could keep everyone updated.

Christine: You know when we were told on December 16th, the day of the Christmas party that there was an issue with the very first CT scan, and even leading up to that with the pericarditis and pneumonia, had it ever crossed your mind that it could be something more serious?

Rod: No, I guess with the pericarditis, because my brother had it a few years before and he communicated with me how he went through it and fully recovered. So, I believed that was all it was and then I had to have those follow up tests on my heart and I had tests previously on my heart and there was no indication of any issues, so I wasn't that worried.

Christine: For me, it felt like we were blind-sided. Earlier in the year I had said to you I felt that this was the start of something much bigger, but it still blindsided us when it came along.

Rod: Yes.

Christine: There was a moment though where you might have thought, and we didn't discuss it at the time, that what if it's worst-case scenario and we refused to use the word death or dying, so we used the terminology 'worst case scenario'. But there was a moment when you said to me, if it was worst case scenario, that you would just tell your brothers to come and get what they wanted from the shed. So, at that point had you been thinking about if it's worst-case scenario?

Rod: Yeah, of course, I did start to think this is going on and on, and the indications from some of the top specialists was that this was suspicious, and remember we still hadn't had the results at that time.

Christine: We googled a lot of it though hadn't we, tumours of the heart?

Rod: Yes, that's right, and if it was what they were indicating we knew that it was quite rare and would be difficult to treat, and plus we didn't know how far it had spread. You start to think, well, if it's spread to other parts of my body, it's going to be difficult to fix it. You start to think I might have to start thinking the worst. They all wanted to go through my shed anyway (laughter), they might as well come and get it while they can.

Christine: Do you think back then there was anything that we had left unspoken between us, that we should have covered together, or do you think we were both skirting around it trying not to talk about worst case scenario?

Rod: I don't think we really discussed it in detail, but we obviously started talking about Wills and ownership of things so that if something happened a lot quicker than we thought, that it would be easier for you and the family to deal with but those sorts of things we gradually started to put them in place anyway.

Christine: So back to when we heard those words "cardiac angiosarcoma", it would have been difficult for you because you were in hospital and I was at Kate's, and that was my greatest fear that they were going to tell us it was that. When you rang me to tell me that, it was like everything going into slow motion and being outside of my body. It felt like I had jumped outside of my body and was watching myself crying in Kate's bedroom. What was that like for you being in the hospital alone and ringing me to tell me that?

Rod: I guess it was softened down a bit for me because I got on quite well with James, the cardiothoracic surgeon, who came and told me about it and confirmed what it was after the surgery and samples. But obviously, at that time, he believed eventually it could be removed, maybe not straight away. But remember those thoughts got squashed after we spoke to Tim and got the next pet scan. Tim definitely didn't soften anything down, he told us this was extremely serious and that really hits home especially, when you don't know what you were in for.

Christine: Were you scared then?

Rod: At that time, I hadn't really read much about it before, and Tim talked about it in a different way from James, who was keen to remove it. Tim doesn't sugar coat anything with his words, as he said, 'it's very rare, serious, don't know a lot about it,' and it's going to be a case of let's see if the chemotherapy he had in mind would work.

Christine: When we spoke to James the next day after diagnosis, and he said to me and Kate that he had seen the tumour and it wasn't resectable because, at that time, it was too big. That must have felt like a blow to you, knowing he couldn't go straight in, and that you would have to have chemo.

Rod: I was still confident that this would have to be the plan for now, move away from James and go ahead with Tim and chemotherapy... have whatever chemo they are going to throw at me to shrink it enough to remove it. I was still positive that we could deal with the chemo. Although I think the chemo is scary too though, because you hear so much about chemo and what it does to people, and that they can't handle it. Tim did tell us he was going to give us some pretty full-on chemo. So, irrespective of how you feel about the tumour, it's another world going into how you are going to deal with the chemo and what it's going to do to you. I was thinking about that, losing my hair, and hearing things about what it does to other people and that sometimes it works and sometimes it doesn't, and you're in the hands of the oncologist and hope that he knows what he's doing.

Christine: Did it feel like being out of control for you? For me, that whole period felt completely out of control... there was nothing about this whole thing that we could control and both of us are very much control freaks. You have a very strong way of doing things yourself, the same as I do. You are very much a planner and methodical thinker, whereas, I too have to know the plan, have to know where we're going and what the future holds. So, for me there was no control, I felt completely in the hands of somebody else and we had to put our whole trust and your life in the hands of someone we didn't really know. What was that like for you?

Rod: It was pretty much exactly the same. We didn't have any control over it, but the only thing I convinced myself over was that the chemo was going to work no matter what. I was going to deal with it and get this thing shrunk enough and get it out. My whole mindset was about getting removed from me later.

Christine: When we talk about mindset, I think that for you it's been huge, this whole journey. yours is always unwavering, whereas mine has been up and down. And it's a lot of trust to put in people. Did you feel we had the best team?

Rod: Yes, absolutely. James was good for us at the time, even though he thought he might not be doing any surgery on me. But, in that really difficult time leading up to the diagnosis, and eventually when he ended up getting the sample himself and then giving us the news about it, he did so with so much consideration for both of us. At the same time, he was the one who contacted Tim because he knew that Tim had some experience with this type of tumour, and both seemed like they were very confident that between them they could come up with a plan. I definitely think we ended up with a really good team of people, and that made me feel more comfortable that they could get it under control.

Christine: I want to talk about unhelpful words, such as keep your chin up, stay positive, the treatment is going to work. My viewpoint is going to be different to yours because as a counsellor I know that they really aren't helpful words. I felt it better if people could just hold space for us and listen to us, because no one at that time knew if it was going to be okay, and it gives people hope when perhaps there might not have been any hope. Not so much now, but in those early days, how did you feel about it when people say, "You've got this Rod, keep your chin up, it's going to work." What goes through your mind when you hear that sort of stuff?

Rod: Well, I don't think I had that many people say that directly to me. Most people were careful about what they said. I don't think I had anyone say, "You've got this," until we started to communicate with posts on social media and we got those good results after the first three months of chemo. Then people started saying things like, "You've got this Keepy, you're really strong." Even though they say it, I don't really think I'm that strong.

Christine: Why would you question that you're not that strong?

Rod: Well I don't think I am; it depends on how they are saying it. People saying you've got this, we knew you could beat it and get on top of it, but they don't know the whole story. We sit there with Tim, and even though it's gone to sleep, all indications are it's going to come back. So even though people are saying those sorts of things, they mean well, but I didn't get a lot of those comments before, so for me it didn't bother me. There were more comments after the third PET scan.

Christine: Did those words make you feel stronger though?

Rod: Yes, they did after that, because I was pretty confident before the third PET scan that we were going to get a good result, and that it had shrunk, and that we were going to get rid of it, but as we know that didn't happen.

Christine: What does it feel like to have cancer in your body, could you actually feel it?

Rod: Not really, I would still have those nights where I would get the full-on coughing fit, which we now know was the tumour irritating my chest lining. It was scary at those times, because I couldn't lie down and get comfortable. But once I started the chemo, the cough and the pain stopped almost straight away, which Tim said he was happy with. But obviously, I had the issues when the chemo started, and I don't really know if that was the cancer or the chemo, and we don't know at what point in that first three months the cancer went to sleep. I don't think anyone would really know that, but I know the cough and the symptoms were very annoying and worrying, and they stopped within the week.

Christine: What is it like watching cancer adverts on TV, knowing you have cancer?

Rod: I don't like watching them, I don't know why. Whenever I see cancer information pop up on Facebook I flick straight over it. I won't read them. But you know there's a lot of sad stuff in amongst all that and down the track, if mine comes back and I end up really sick from it, that's different. But at the moment, reading and continuously seeing stuff about cancer or when we are watching a movie where someone has cancer, I don't like watching it.

Christine: I guess it's hard, because prior to your diagnosis we would have watched it even though it made us feel uncomfortable. Whereas now it's like this is us.

Rod: Yes, it could be me, which is hard to watch and think about.

Christine: Even though we know that TV shows exaggerate, the reality is it still must be hard.

Rod: Any type of advertising on cancer or through the media, I just flick straight over it.

Christine: Do you think that a bit of being in denial, it's not happening to me or is it I just don't want to see it because that is me?

Rod: I just don't want to see it… I don't want to be confronted with it and don't want to be like that person.

Christine: I fell into the trap of asking you are you okay, which as a counsellor I know is wrong and I bite my tongue every time it comes out of my mouth. But every time I see you touch your chest or hear you cough or groan, my fear kicks in, and I ask you are you okay. What is that like for you being constantly asked how you are doing?

Rod: (Laughter) It frustrates me, (more laughter). Like I said before, you question at times, you have a cry and thinking about it, that's the same. I clearly understand that's your way.

Christine: It's the fear of losing you that makes me cry.

Rod: I recognise that it's fear, but under my breath I'm saying "Well, I'm frigging alright." It's like it doesn't really bother me, but whenever I go to touch a part of my body and you go "are you okay, are you okay?"... and you do it quite a lot, then I'm thinking to myself, I'm pretty sure if I wasn't, I would be going to tell you.

Christine: Well, that's where I'm not so sure, I think you do hide stuff from me and for me it is purely fear based. I live from scan to scan, in fear. We do okay for the first few weeks, months, then as it gets closer, and I know we have a scan coming, and I get scanxiety again and the fear comes back. I don't think that's ever going to go away, that's how our life is now, our new norm. But I am trying to find a different way to communicate with you which is hard because sometimes I get angry with you. When you cut yourself, I get angry with you because you frigging know your susceptible to infection and I get angry that you're not taking care of yourself.

Rod: Hmmm (laughter from both of us).

I decided to leave the interview at this point. I could see that Rod was getting tired and I was actually surprised how open he had been with me.

THE POWER OF POSITIVE MINDSET

Positive psychology was, for many years, frowned upon as we went down the route of clinical interventions and medication. However, over the last decade, there has been a subtle shift back to positive psychology and holistic therapy. I believe in the power of the mind and its ability to communicate with the body, which can then enable the right conditions to fight illness, disease, anxiety, and improve overall emotional happiness.

I really wanted to write this chapter about Rod's mindset, along with my own. As in an earlier chapter, I mentioned that I found myself in a dark place the moment that life started to stabilise for us. You might think this odd; if things were improving, so then should my mindset. But as I wrote about in that chapter, my nervous system had been in fight or flight for so long it no longer knew how to regulate itself, and my brain started to struggle to make sense of this change in our circumstances.

There is some truth in the saying that "who you surround yourself with will reflect and rub off onto you". Surrounding yourself with people who are fearful and negative will increase the energy of fear and negativity in your own life. On the flip side, surrounding yourself with positive and uplifting people will increase your energy and emotional well-being. I used to teach this in workshops and know this theory well, yet I still went down the dark rabbit hole myself.

When I realised I was sliding down that dark hole and the effect it was also having on Rod, I knew something had to change, and quickly. Luckily, I had the tools to pull myself back from the darkness along with the support of my friends, most of whom are highly spiritual as well. But I also recognised how important it was for me to stay there and not slide back.

In a moment of synchronicity, my friend, Jodi, told me about a two-day workshop she was attending on meditation and mindset. I looked at the details and without hesitation booked my place at the workshop. Whilst the workshop wasn't anything new to me - I know a great deal about the power of mindset - it did give me the prod I needed to get back on track. I came home excited with the knowledge that, once again, Rod and I together as a collective energy, can assist with the healing process.

I'm not suggesting that it's possible to stay in a high vibrational state all the time. We are human beings who experience a wide range of emotions. What I am suggesting is that we take the time to honour where we are in this present moment, and if in that moment it feels heavy and sad, sit there with it for a few minutes or hours, then try to move through it, get up and move, do something you enjoy. As a somatic therapist, one thing I have learnt is that movement is the key to releasing energy. If you were to picture yourself sad or fearful, the first response in your body is to hunch your shoulders and tighten your jaw. Your breathing becomes shallower and your body contracts, and often anxiety or panic sets in. This is when movement becomes helpful. Try to get up and allow your chest to expand, stretch your arms out to your sides or pull your shoulders back, tilt your head more upright to open your chest, do some deep breathing, focus on releasing the tension in your jaw and allow your body to regulate. Shaking off your tension and anxiety is another tool I use. Literally, shaking parts of your body gently. Shaking your arms, hands and legs all helps to release negative trapped energy.

It's also important to reach out to others for support. Additionally, practicing gratitude helps me, even when the thought of gratitude is the furthest thing from my mind. There is always something to be grateful for, sometimes simply the warmth of your pet or a flower you love. I often look around and scan my surroundings and find something to focus on. I am a cloud gazer and when I do this, along with taking a few long and slow, deep breaths, I find my nervous system can regulate itself relatively quickly.

Rod's attitude through this journey has been amazing. I'm so very proud of the way he is handling this. His unwavering belief that he will heal and how he gets on with life is something to be acknowledged. When he started treatment, I was worried about him getting nausea. I asked him about this, and he said, "I'm just telling myself I'm not going to get that side effect." If he feels a slight lean towards it, he tells his body it's not happening, and he uses distraction as his key. I find it astonishing that he can control his body like that. To me, that's is a sign of true determination and strength.

The same can be said for the nurses in the chemo suite. When you arrive, they are all so cheerful, even though every patient they have is fighting some form of cancer and are more than likely filled with fear. They do their jobs day in and day out, often run off their feet, understaffed, tired and hungry. But they never let it show and their infectious moods lighten up what is a horrible situation.

I'll take a moment here, as I'm writing this book, to give huge gratitude and acknowledgement to the medical professionals who work with cancer care and treatment.

I often refer to our journey as living our lives alongside cancer. I was watching a documentary when I first heard this terminology, and it changed the whole way I think about a cancer diagnosis. Rod's cancer diagnosis is only a small part of who we are as a couple, and how we live our lives. Neither of us let this overwhelm us anymore to the point of feeling stuck and completely out of control. There are still times when I am fearful and overwhelmed, but once again for me, the key is not staying in that space too long. Whilst this doesn't mean that we don't take Rod's diagnosis seriously, this rare and aggressive cancer has entered and become part of our lives, but we do have the choice to decide how much of a part it plays. As a couple, there are many parts to our lives, and each day we make the commitment to each other, our relationship, and our souls to do the things we enjoy and love.

One thing we decided to do early on this journey was to have cancer free days. This means spending time together, going on a date or being out with friends and family where the talk of cancer is not welcome. Whilst it is constantly in the back of our minds, we have found this highly beneficial to remember we are also a couple in a relationship, and not just someone who has cancer and the partner of someone who has cancer. Prioritising our relationship above the cancer diagnosis is something we constantly work on.

We are truly living our lives alongside his cancer diagnosis, and I love it when I hear others say, "We are living with cancer, not dying from it." While Rod is strong and functioning, we are continuing to go about our lives and undertake our plans that we have for the future. In an earlier chapter I wrote about how Rod found it difficult to let go of work and see the benefits of short trips and outings, coupled with rest when he needs to support his body. But as time goes on, this is no longer an issue for us. At one stage, I thought our chances of travel were out of the question. Rod, on the other hand, had full faith that this would occur, and I am extremely grateful that we still have this as part of our plan.

OUR RELATIONSHIP & MY OWN SELF CARE

Rod and I have changed a lot as a couple through this journey. We've learnt things about each other that we didn't recognise before. I've certainly seen a different side to him, and him me. I'm not sure if it was always there or whether we hid it better before, and now it's coming to light given his cancer diagnosis. Those words "you have cancer," can certainly change your perspective on life. It can be a "well, what have I got to lose" attitude, so I might as well take the mask off and expose the real me. I'm not saying this is every couple's experience, and sometimes we aren't even aware of the masks we wear with our partners. But, for me, it was an interesting reflection on myself and him.

I've learnt that I meltdown quickly, or in Layla's words, "Nanna's having a tantrum." Rod has certainly recognised when those moments are arising. He can see the warning signs and picks up on my signals quickly. We have had many occasions where we have been out and my anxiety levels have started to rise, and I feel like I have to get out of there. Particularly, when it comes to being around lots of people and noise. I think I have always been affected by other's energy and if there's too much in one space, I feel my breathing gets shallower and my shoulders start to tense, and often I will get a headache.

Now, I have added another step in that process, I run… I must get away, and my body goes straight into flight mode. There was one occasion in a roadhouse on the way home from one of Rod's many tests, where we stopped to get something to eat. There were busloads of children all travelling back from a trip away, and they were everywhere in the roadhouse. The noise was horrific; I walked straight into them and instantly my flight mode kicked in. In that moment I felt like I couldn't breathe; I started pulling at my clothing which felt very tight, even though it wasn't. I started looking for an escape route in the building. The noise I heard sounded amplified, my body was heating up and I found myself wanting to scream. Rod took one look at me and said, "Get out of here, I'll get the food and bring it out to the car." While he laughed about it with me later, I could see on his face at the time that he was thinking, "OK, here we go, she's about to burst, I need to step in," and I'm so grateful that he can read me in those moments.

I used to believe that Rod and I had a lot in common, and maybe it was easier when we were both working full time and only spending a few hours a day with each other. When you are thrown together (albeit, by our own choice) twenty-four hours a day, seven days a week, you really start to notice things you wouldn't have before. I have thought about this many times and I can see how couples often end up divorced, when one or both retire. One day Rod was heading off to work each morning at 6:20 a.m., and I would be getting on with my routine of walking the dog and working, and not seeing each other until 6:00 that night. Then, in a split second, here we were spending all our time at home or running to and from treatments and appointments. This was such an upheaval for us both and has taken some adjusting to, which has certainly given me a new perspective on relationships.

Self-care sounds selfish when it's not you faced with a cancer diagnosis. It felt like I had no right to think about myself, when Rod was fighting for his life. My life became consumed with supporting him and all my own routines went out the window. The days when I'm exhausted or ill and Rod does things for me, I feel guilty. I think to myself, *he's the one who's ill, I shouldn't be complaining about how I'm feeling. My pain or illness is nowhere near as bad as what he's going through.* In those moments I used to shut down and try to hide what was going on for me.

It can be a whole different dynamic when you are trying to balance not only your relationship as partners, but also the element of caregiver/patient, especially in the early days. Many caregivers I know often put their own self-care on the back burner until they become emotionally and physically exhausted. I was no different, I had put my own self-care on the back burner. One of my friends asked me one day what I was doing for me. I looked at her blankly and defensively said, "I'm meditating, journaling and resting, I feel that's enough." She gently asked again what I was doing for me? I stopped and reflected more on this and answered, "Nothing really."

I get told it's my journey too, and I do acknowledge this, but I'm the one who's going to live and there goes the guilt again. *Rod might die and I'm going to live.* I often wonder how he feels about that. Does he feel resentful? I certainly wouldn't blame him if he did. I can't even start to imagine what that thought would be like for him. So, with this in mind, self-care felt selfish. Yet deep down I knew that if I was going to be strong for him, if I was to be able to fully support him, I needed to look after myself.

I also find it interesting that I can talk about self-care with clients yet couldn't allow myself the same. I reflect on what self-care looked like for me. Is it about honouring my own needs, doing things that bring me joy? I used to run baths for Rod or watch him run one for himself; putting magnesium flakes into his bath whilst enviously wishing I could have one too, but feeling that I didn't deserve one. Prior to the cancer diagnosis I wouldn't have hesitated to run myself a bath or ask Rod to make me a cup of tea or do something for me. Subconsciously, by not looking after my own self-care, I was turning him into a patient and taking away his independence and ability to be my partner, as well as de-valuing my own self-worth in this relationship.

Partnerships are about give and take - a balance of giving and receiving - but when illness strikes that balance gets thrown out of whack. It was important for us to function as a couple rather than patient and caregiver, and I knew I needed to even us back up. So, I started treating him like my husband again. I started sharing with him when I felt ill, I spoke about my aches and pains. I would ask him to make me a cup of tea. Rod loves cooking outside on his barbecue, so I started asking him if he would cook dinner or go to the shops to buy our groceries. I was giving him back his purpose as a partner and restoring my own self-care.

Now don't get me wrong, our relationship is solid and resilient, but just like everyone else in this situation, we are still navigating our way through this new normal and it can come with frustrations that occasionally spill over into our relationship. Living from scan to scan in three monthly blocks, is also a relationship roller-coaster. This has me thinking what if every relationship had to think in terms of three months at a time. Would people make more of an effort with each other? For me, it feels like we are re-negotiating the terms of our marriage with each scan cycle. Waiting to see what comes next and what we can achieve together in these next three months. It is hard to look too far into the future when there is a cloud of uncertainty hanging over our heads. It's why we call it "living our lives alongside cancer," not letting it define us as a couple whilst trying desperately to remain partners, not patient and caregiver, or someone who has cancer and the partner of someone who has cancer.

Some days are easier than others. If Rod is doing well and not so tired it can be easy to forget that he has a cancer diagnosis. Life feels normal for a short while. He often pushes himself hard to get things he wants done and then goes into what I call his crash and burn days. On these crash and burn days he's tired and sleeps in longer than me. I find him a bit withdrawn, the pain from the side effects of treatment showing on his face, and it's in those moments the harsh reality smacks me in the face again.

We often get frustrated with each other. I research, read and watch lots of videos on how to beat cancer, trying to engage Rod in the process, usually to no avail. This is my way of trying to control and fix the situation. But for Rod, I believe the power of his own mind is all he needs. I sometimes feel that there are three in our relationship now. Rod, me, and Tim, our oncologist, as neither of us will make any changes to our plans until we have talked it over with Tim. I once asked him if he would like to see a cancer coach or have a consult with a naturopath who might be able to help strengthen his immune system while he is still having chemo. The answer I got was, "No thanks, I'm happy with Tim". I laughed about this with him, as I responded that "I wasn't asking you to divorce Tim, I just thought maybe a consult with a naturopath or coach who could help with exercise or nutrition might help." Tim and his team have become a huge part of our life and this is something Rod and I laugh about when I ask him, "And what do you think Tim would say to this?"

I also recognise I have this new role to play in our relationship, one where I must remember or remind Rod to do something or take something. I had heard the words chemo brain before, but I can fully understand what it means now. The treatment has left Rod a little fuzzy at times and often he doesn't remember where he has put things, or conversations that we have had. Prior to starting treatment, Rod's memory was amazing. He could recall the smallest detail from years ago, especially if it was during one of our few arguments, repeating my words back to me.

When it comes to food or supplements, I just put them in front of him and he will take them. But if I let them slide, then so does he. Something I am used to as a counsellor with understanding humans and our ability to change, it can be hard to maintain. New habits or long-term behaviours take a great deal of effort and energy to achieve. Couple that with chemo brain, and it's a whole new dynamic. You may be thinking that it's not my responsibility to do all of this, but Rod and I are a partnership and when he isn't able to do something or maintain something, especially when dealing with treatment and the stress of the diagnosis, then I believe it's my role to step up.

In the moments when I do get frustrated with him for not looking after himself, I vent to my friends, Vicki, Michelle and Jodi, who patiently hear me out, and then I manage to put it to one side and get back on with life. I am so grateful to have them all, as well as many others in my life who are my support team. Whereas Rod internalises and often keeps his thoughts to himself, even though I see his frustration with me. Not being able to express his frustration or thoughts with me, he often retreats to his projects, putting some space between us. The counsellor in me finds this difficult and I'm often thinking of different ways to broach subjects with him - he certainly keeps me on my toes.

I believe the one, most important thing to have in maintaining your relationship, is external support. There appears to be so much emphasis about being honest with each other, being able to tell each other everything without fear of repercussions or judgement. But in my opinion, even as a former relationship counsellor, some of our thoughts can be harmful and detrimental to the person and the relationship. I advocate for being discerning on how much you share with your partner, and using a journal or talking to someone you trust who can handle your thoughts carefully and safely.

I'm slowly getting back to doing the things I love, and we have started doing things separately at home. For me, that's writing and de-cluttering our house. De-cluttering is truly good for the soul and refreshing to the energy within the home. I often ask myself in the morning *what can I do to support myself today, what does my body require from me today, or how can I show my soul that I care and show up for myself today?* I often write these answers in my journal to reinforce how important I am in this world as well. For Rod, it's small projects, things that he had been getting around to for years. I feel that in some ways I've grown and evolved more than Rod. When I look back, I realise he's really not doing anything differently than he used to, except for being kinder to himself and knowing his own limits. Yet, here I am, feeling like a completely new version of myself.

Some of the activities we used to do together, now leave me feeling unsatisfied. I often wonder if that's because I live with a "limited time outlook," whereas Rod lives with an "all the time in the world" perspective. I'm a neat freak and his world is disorganised chaos. We are still trying to work that balance out. I'm a planner and like to have things laid out well in advance, often ready to go out hours before we need to and Rod's a last-minute man, which means he is running around at the last minute while I sit there holding back my frustration.

Now, I'm not suggesting that we have absolutely nothing in common, but we have certainly noticed our differences. We still share the same sense of humor, the things we find amusing. We love visiting new places and experiencing life together. We laugh and tease each other just as much as we used to. I'm the first person he rings to tell me some news he has heard, and he is still the person I want to come home to everyday. Rod loves his boat and his fishing. I just love the ocean, so while he fishes I sit on the beach and soak up the rawness and beauty that the water holds. We both love our bikes and going for a ride, often turning it into a date with riding to lunch or dinner. Our relationship is also about compromise. Rod booked a concert for us to attend as a surprise because he knows I like the singer, and I booked a day at the races and to go to the football with him, even though I'm not keen on football.

There's a sense of belonging within our relationship, something to protect and honour. We are proud of each other's achievements in life and are not afraid to show that to the world. We are each other's biggest cheerleaders. We have cancer free days which we both feel is important to maintaining our connection with each other, just as it's important to remember that we each have individual needs and wants. We still dream of a future together, however long that might be, although it might be a slightly different vision to the one we have but it's one we both hold onto.

We often spend our morning over our coffee, sitting quietly with each other. While Rod checks on sports news and flicks through social media, before I start work I write in my journal, pull an oracle card and reflect on what messages come through. I often ask him if he would like an oracle card, and patiently indulging me, he shuffles and then chooses one. When I ask him what question he asked for guidance on, he often replies with whether a particular horse will win an upcoming race, or whether his footy team will win. This makes me laugh as I try to explain to him that oracle cards are a tool for reflection and inner wisdom, not for predicting the future of his sporting interests.

During the day, he tries to have an hour's rest while I read or work on my writing, before going about our different activities again. In the evenings we create space for each other; that space where we come together over dinner and watch a TV show or movie. It's a calm space and an environment that fosters connection. I light candles, have soft lighting throughout the house and everything from the day starts to slow down to a gentle pace, where all our differences in that moment and the days stresses are forgotten.

But I feel the biggest growth to come from this journey as a couple, is tolerance and kindness. Tolerance for our differences, learning who we are as we evolve as a couple and individuals. Tolerance not only for Rod, but also for myself. Showing kindness in the way we treat each other, being gentle in those moments of high stress, each checking in with the other to see how we're doing. Smiling at each other first thing in the morning, and last thing at night. Stopping what we are doing throughout the day to listen to each other when we want to share our news. Our commitment to each other and our relationship is as strong as ever, and while he continues to drive me nuts with his messiness each day, I am eternally grateful for the man whom I call my husband. Whilst our future is still unknown, we continue to enjoy every day we have together filled with love, laughter, and searching for those rainbows.

IN CONCLUSION: WHO AM I NOW?

Who am I now? This is a question I have asked myself many times since we started this journey in December 2022. I've had many identities and roles in this world. I'm a wife, mother, grandmother, sister, friend, colleague, business owner, counsellor, somatic trauma therapist and healer. Like many others, I've often linked my identity to my work and my business. In our hometown I'm known as Soulful C. But when Rod was diagnosed with cancer, I put my business on hold, and that got me thinking, *who am I now?* I'm still all those things I was before, but with my focus being completely on Rod and his journey I wondered where Soulful C had gone. I had seemed to have lost a part of myself and my identity in this world.

I always thought I pretty much had it all together. Like most humans I have my flaws, my insecurities, and my own quirky personality. I knew what I wanted from life and wasn't afraid to go out and get it or change track if I needed to. If you were to ask my friends, they would all say I can adapt quickly to new situations and circumstances, and take it all in my stride with ease and grace. But all that changed the day we heard those words "Rod, you have a suspicious mass". Those words altered my direction and perspective on life instantly. I watched myself shrink to what I thought was a shadow of my former self.

People kept telling me *you're so strong, you have such a positive attitude,* but in my mirror, I hardly recognised myself. Not only had I linked my identity to my work and business, but I had also linked it to Rod. Being his wife is something I'm so proud of. I threw myself into supporting him so much, that I felt like we had melded into one.

When we got the amazing news that the cancer had gone to sleep and the tumour had shrunk, life started to stabilise. It was then that my role of support wasn't needed as much. Rod was feeling better with the tumour no longer pressing heavily against his heart. The chemo side effects were nowhere near as bad, and he was feeling stronger in himself.

So, who am I now and what lies ahead for me? At the time of writing this book, I have returned to my business, although these days it looks very different than it did at the start of this journey. My focus is on supporting others who are going through a similar journey to my own in a holistic and soul aligned way.

But who is the real Christine behind the name Soulful C?

I know I am not the person I was when we started this journey. I've grown so much both spiritually and emotionally. I've had to deal with this trauma the best way I know how. I have a side to me that can meltdown quickly, as I've talked about in previous chapters. I have found that I need to feel in control and when I don't, I retreat to my journal to help me process what is really going on in this moment. I wrote about our holiday odyssey but in reality, it was just as much of a spiritual odyssey for me. I connected back to myself in a much deeper way than I had before.

I made the commitment to myself at the start of 2024, that I would honour myself and my needs a bit more this year. We were in for a long haul, and I needed to not l(o)ose myself in the process. What this looks like, I'm still working through, but I know that a healing retreat is definitely in the cards, finally getting to visit my friend, Vicki, and see her new home, reconnecting with others I've unintentionally ignored these past twelve months, and I've joined various writer's groups. Through this journey, I've found that I love writing far more than I first realised. Writing this book has helped me to process my own pain and set me on my own healing journey. This is so much different to writing in my journal, which I still do every morning, asking my soul what it requires from me each day and how I can support myself better. I would never have imagined, back in December 2022, that I would be sitting here today writing a book about my journey supporting Rod through a cancer diagnosis, so I guess that makes me a writer. Writing will be something I will continue, long after this book is completed, and I already have an outline for the next one.

I've found a strength and resilience that I didn't know I had. I've discovered the strength to show up in my most vulnerable moments and do so with a passion, where I don't want anyone to feel that what they are going through is not normal or that they are weak. I'm deeply spiritual and not afraid to show this to the world, which scares some people because I use energy healing, sound bowls and oracle cards. I laugh at this because I recognise this is their own fear of something they don't understand. I meditate and listen to both etherical and country music, two complete opposites. I'm still all the things I used to be, with a different flavour to me now.

I'm more authentic with family and friends, no longer afraid of judgement. I'm still on a path of self-discovery, unlocking parts of me I didn't know existed. Aspects of my soul have suddenly appeared and I'm embracing this new me. I recognise that I am so much more than an individual soul, I'm more deeply connected now to others and the Universe. I see aspects of myself in others and them in me. I'm a better partner for Rod, we have grown together through this journey and have a deeper connection than ever, even through our frustrations. This chapter of my life has shown me that all my years of training in counselling and trauma therapy, along with energy healing, have provided me with the tools to work my way through this.

I am, and always will be, eternally grateful to the medical staff who follow this difficult path to help research, treat or cure cancer and to the cancer nurses who give themselves tirelessly, day in, day out, and are some of the most beautiful souls I have ever met. But the real hero in this journey is my husband, Rod. I am so proud of how he is handling this diagnosis and his strength and determination to not let this overcome him. He does this with such grace and humour, and he is truly an inspiration.

I hope that by reading about our experience and my personal reflections, you recognise parts of yourself in here, that you become gentler with yourself, realise that you are stronger than you think, and that you, too, can search for and find your rainbow when faced with adversity.

I have reflected much on the journey that Rod and I have undertaken through his cancer diagnosis, who we were prior, who we are as a couple and who I am now. It seemed through the trauma and pain, I acknowledge how much I have grown as a soul, and I wish you, the reader, much love and healing on your own journey - Christine

ACKNOWLEDGMENTS

There are a number of people who have inspired me and helped me through the process of writing and publishing this book and I wanted to take a moment to acknowledge and honour their contribution:

Assoc Prof. Dr. Tim Clay - Medical Oncologist, and his team for their care, support, and endless commitment to their clients.

The cancer nurses at the Bendat Cancer Centre, St John of God Hospital Subiaco WA - who make the process so much easier.

My dearest friends - Vicki, Michelle, Jodi, Kay, Tarryn and Julie, for picking me up off the floor when I've stumbled and holding me always with their love and support.

My fellow group members in the Facebook group, Cardiac Angiosarcoma Patient and Family Support Group - who take time out of their lives to share research and support each other in the most vulnerable of times.

ABOUT THE AUTHOR

Christine is a professional Counsellor, Somatic Trauma Therapist and Holistic Wellness Practitioner living in the picturesque Southwest Town of Collie Western Australia.

Christine is passionate about supporting others to feel emotional relief, find clarity, confidence and calm in their own lives. Having experienced her own fair share of trauma over the years from domestic violence, to losing family members in horrific circumstances and recovering from cervical cancer herself, it came as a shock when in 2022 her husband Rod was diagnosed with an extremely rare and aggressive cancer.

Through this vulnerable and honest reflection, Christine shares with you how her professional training and spiritual beliefs have helped her to find the strength and courage to move through the trauma that a cancer diagnosis of someone you love can bring and how important it is to honour your own journey in this moment.

www.ingramcontent.com/pod-product-compliance
Lightning Source LLC
Chambersburg PA
CBHW051450290426
44109CB00016B/1703